Stay Sober and Save the World

the Cave Woman Way

Ellen Archer

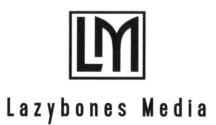

Lazybones Media

Stay Sober and Save the World the Cave Woman Way

Lazybones Media

Paperback ISBN: 979-8-9857567-0-8

PRINTED IN THE UNITED STATES OF AMERICA

Preface

About Cave Woman and Me

With only a notebook at hand and raw with prickly emotions, I wondered, *If I could talk with anyone who ever existed, who would I choose?* I thought of people who lived in healthy communities, who relied on each other's wisdom and practical know-how. That's when I opened to a new page and wrote "Dear Cave Woman" for the first time.

I imagined she'd been watching humanity since prehistoric times. I imagined she knew what would set humanity back on the right track. Back to cooperation and kindness as our main social skills. Back to healing from trauma and pain as daily practices. Back to knowing how to live as humans with more creativity, free from abuse.

Being early in recovery, I only managed a few pages of curse words, but I felt a little better. I started to write to Cave Woman more often, and eventually, my journals turned into *Stay Sober and Save the World the Cave Woman Way.*

We're all in recovery for something. Recovery needn't be a slog. Healing can be fun, even hilarious. Cave Woman taught me to lighten up, play more, and find a bit more ease one letter at a time.

Dedication

To my mom for spinning her magic. We did so well together. You are a big part of this. I believe you now.

And to my husband for being a giant among men and for his love, humor, and inexplicable support.

Why do People Have Addictions?

Dear Cave Woman,

Why do people have addictions?

Let's start with a bit of background. In my community, we relied on each other to remain stable and resilient like a hive of honeybees.

We supported each other, completely and unconditionally. My entire being—my senses, my intuition, my body—craved and was nurtured by this wholeness, by my hive, by a honeyed love that filled in all the crevices.

We supported each other's strengths and offset any weaknesses. It felt amazing to be a part of my hive, like being wildly in love, and you're missing that. You're missing the protection a hive provides within a flourishing ecosystem. The loss can feel irreparable when you think living like a lone bee is your only safe option. Separate-

ness creates a vacuum inside you, and stopgap measures like addictions arise.

No one consciously chooses addiction. The loss of cohesive wise communities proliferated addiction. Addiction is an unconscious attempt to fill an inconceivable void.

Because very few humans live in a healthy community like mine, you won't find one to join. But you can use my community, the hive of my heart, as a metaphor to become a whole human being.

Your beehive needs a few repairs. However, mending the rips and tears causes all your resources to focus, once again, on protecting the queen. With a shored-up hive, you'll align with the guidance that you truly crave.

As you sync up with people actively repairing their own hearts, the protection you gain will leave you less vulnerable to those who would steal your honey.

Enter my cave. Let your eyes adjust to the dark. Then follow the map of your heart to an ancient lineage ready to bid you welcome.

Chapter 1

Frozen North

We live in a cave inside a cave. My boyfriend, Cole, and I live in the basement apartment, caretaking a ski home in exchange for free rent. The house sits up against a mountain, hidden from the sun seven months a year. We also both worked second jobs with demanding clients, which consumed our lives.

We only meant to stay a year, two at most. Ten years later, we're finally leaving for good. Disentangling ourselves from multiple jobs left us parting from more than we'd anticipated. We're moving to Haiti for a new job that can make a big difference in people's lives.

I'm so excited about our new adventure I can't sleep, but I rarely sleep on nights I don't drink. Dawn marks a clean start, and I've decided to quit drinking once and for all. I've made this decision many times before, but I know starting a whole new life will give me the impetus to make quitting stick.

I hate winter, I don't ski, and I'm anxious to leave. I'm worried a lot lately. I'm anxious to leave this town. I look at the clock: 4:00 a.m.

I'm ready to go, so I nudge Cole with my foot a few times to wake him up.

"Are you awake?" I whisper loudly.

"I think so," Cole says with his eyes still closed.

"I'm going to shower now. Can we leave once I'm ready?"

"Might as well," he concedes.

Cole and I finished packing the car last night. We put our belongings in storage and pared down to two bags each.

We take showers and put the last remaining suitcase in the car. With Cole's precious coffee maker in storage, we stop at a convenience store. Coffee for Cole and tea for me.

Back in the car, we drive into a wavering west wind. Dark snow clouds cap the steep, black mountains like a freezer jammed with frost.

One regret chases me. If we drive quickly enough, maybe I can shake it loose. I just need to keep going and concentrate on a more useful future.

On top of our caretaking duties, I worked as a marketing researcher and then drank to relax and forget about work in the evening. As a caretaker for several homes in the area, Cole was permanently on call. We rarely left town. Cole turns off his cell phone and ceremoniously tosses it in the backseat. He whistles, and I cheer.

The sky lightens and I want to feel free, but I don't. For a moment, my one regret makes me want to turn around. My chest grows hot with worry, and I wonder if karma is real. I almost say out loud I have to go back. Instead, I stifle the thought by pushing my hand against my mouth.

I made a painful sacrifice, but I'll work hard to help people and make it all worthwhile. We'd always wanted to make a difference in the world, and we're grabbing our chance, maybe the only one we'll ever have.

We'll stay in Phoenix for a month or so, coordinate with our contacts, and await the final plans for our trip. We picked Phoenix because of the warm weather and because a friend told us we could find a month-to-month rental if we needed to stay longer than our budget allowed for a hotel. We'll leave our car at our friend's house.

Cole will need to finish his coffee before he can talk. I turn on the radio, but the news story annoys me, so I turn it off.

Driving away feels like our rocket has launched and we've not yet reached the smooth edge beyond Earth's orbit. I just have to hold on and endure the uncertainty until new possibilities become real.

I feel vacant without the sound of the radio and turn the news back on.

Light snow begins to fall, and wind forms the snow into white snakes that slither along the highway. I hope the storm doesn't become a full-blown blizzard before we turn south and head away from winter forever. I'll feel better once we're in a warmer climate.

Gravity

Four hours later, we notice a large black bag by the side of the road. We slow down and look in shock at a body bag. A metal zipper with large teeth runs along the top. What looked like tall, dried grass near the bag focuses into a human arm sticking straight up, pale and unmoving.

My stomach does a backflip, and I grab Cole's arm to steady myself. We look at each other in disbelief.

Cole begins to slow down and pull over.

"Don't stop. It might be a trap," I say.

"Sil, we have to stop."

"I know. I know. But not here," I say quickly.

He shakes his head slightly at my paranoia but keeps going.

Cole, raised in a large catholic family in a polite small town, remains trusting and self-sacrificing. A ten-year stint in NYC left me suspicious and wary despite a childhood in the naïve suburbs.

We note the mile marker and veer into a gravel pullout, and Cole calls the police.

They don't seem to believe Cole, and he has to repeat himself several times.

I keep a keen eye on the rear-view mirror.

As we pull away, I shudder and say, "Holy crap. What the hell?" This isn't the smooth lift-off I'd envisioned.

"How in the world…?" Cole shakes his head and looks at me for an answer.

"I can't begin to imagine how a body in a body bag ends up by the side of a highway. I really can't," I say.

Cole picks up where I left off, "And with an arm sticking out. I can't even think of a joke." Cole's soft-spoken nature hides a brilliant and quick wit if you listen closely.

A quiet, eerie gravity replaces the elation of leaving the long winters and long work hours. I rummage through the backseat for a book on CD.

"Dinosaur National Monument, next exit," Cole reads on a sign and starts to slow down. "Want to take a look?"

"I've wanted to see the petroglyphs for years," I say.

"It'll add several hours of driving, but maybe it will help get the body bag off our minds," Cole offers.

"Maybe," I answer.

"We'll have to get a hotel closer than the one we reserved in Arizona for tonight."

"Okay. Want me to cancel our reservation?"

"Yeah, change it to tomorrow. Let's take our time; stop and look at rocks and stuff."

"Good idea," I say cheerfully and pull my phone from the console. Still, I can't help wondering if the body bag portends a bad omen or highlights the nagging regret I feel. If it's both, I might as well throw myself off a cliff.

Short Windy Hike

About two hours later, we turn off the highway and follow the signs to the petroglyphs. The high desert spreads endlessly, stippled with red mesas like a painting but without mountains crowding every square inch. The first petroglyphs aren't too far off the highway and only a short walk from the parking area. I'm relieved. Since deciding to stop drinking for our new adventure, I'm feeling unsteady, and I'm not up for a long hike. Despite my fresh start, I'm still wobbly and shaky.

On the short windy hike, the rocks in my stomach multiply and pile up in my chest, increasing my anxiety. I'm afraid it'll get worse, and my worry will spread to Cole. I need to stay upbeat. I decide to drink tonight and instantly feel better. Alcohol will keep doubts at bay. A tiny thrill replaces the dread in my stomach, and my pace picks up.

Cole points out big cat tracks alongside the trail. "They're fresh," he says.

A chill ripples down my back. "Do you think it's still around?"

"I wouldn't be surprised if it was watching us right now," Cole says, and I don't know if he's joking or not.

"I'd rather be food for a mountain lion than end up in a body bag by the side of the road. At least I'd provide a meal," I say. I'd come pre-marinated in wine, I joke to myself.

We walk on, listening to the stubborn wind sweep the canyons clean. I scan the terrain for wild hungry cats.

Cole stops and points to a drawing etched in the burnt umber rock face just above us. I would have passed right by the subtle stone carving and not noticed anything. We scrabble up the slight incline to get closer and lean my knees against a boulder just below the drawing.

Much more prominent than the other figures, the woman carved in the center seems to be decked out in ceremonial garb. I wonder if she's a goddess or a real person, a leader, or someone's beloved mother. Like my beloved mom.

One hand reaches into a swirl surrounded by short rays, an image I've doodled in notebooks many times. I want to understand, to comprehend the significance. I wonder if they sell wine at gas stations in Utah. I might need to find a liquor store. My focus shifts, and for a moment, she's looking right at me, eye to eye. I wait for a bolt-of-lightning insight, but nothing comes, and instead, I feel numb. The disconnect irritates me.

A cold wind kicks up the loose soil, and Cole and I both wipe the nippy dirt from our faces. Nausea blankets me in a dizzying wave. I hold my face in my hands to steady myself. The tall red rocks have captured the sun's heat, so I touch my cheek and hands to the boulder and absorb the warmth. I imagine ancient artists standing here, and I hear faint voices, muffled and indistinct, like the voices I heard as a kid during a high fever. My eardrums vibrate like a bass guitar. I can't make out a single word. I shiver.

I feel a panic attack approaching, so I sink cross-legged to the dirt. I pick up a few small rocks, so Cole thinks I'm looking for fossils. My face goes numb and my eyes follow an invisible swirl. I shut my eyes to stop the motion. I feel like my soul is slowly giving up on me and sneaking away through the top of my head. I don't want Cole to think I'm having a panic attack, so I keep combing through rocks. A thought or notion starts to form, something I'm not sure I want to know, so I hold my breath and only allow tiny sips of air. I scratch H E L P into the tan, hard-packed dirt, which I quickly erase, so Cole won't think I've lost my mind.

"I'm cold. You ready to leave?" I complain to Cole.

I don't linger. In nature, in museums, in restaurants. Once I'm done, I'm ready to leave.

"We just got here," Cole repeats, probably for the ten-thousandth time since we first met. He could linger in canyons, deserts, or forests and explore for hours.

"Fifteen minutes?" I offer in what feels like a compromise. "And we'll go see more petroglyphs, okay?"

"Okay," he says and shrugs.

Go Ahead Without Me

I stay in the car at our next stop as Cole wanders the lonely canyons. I find the audiobook under the front seat and turn on the car periodically to keep the battery charged. I hate silence. Cole finally returns. We head out and stop at a gas station just outside Dinosaur National Monument. I buy a notebook with a cartoon dinosaur on the cover. To appease my craving for alcohol until we stop for the night, I buy a soda and a big bag of potato chips. After we find a motel, I can look for a proper liquor store to stock up for the evening.

At 7:20 p.m., we pull into yet another western-themed tourist town and look for a motel. Since I decided to drink at the petroglyphs, the impatience turned my neck and shoulder to stone. To help pass the time, we rattled off western decor we will not miss like neon cowboys, neon cowboy boots, neon dancing cowgirls, hitching posts, antler chandeliers, and all the wooden bears and noble Native Americans that seemed more like the spoils of genocide than an honorific.

There isn't much traffic, and we find a motel conveniently located next to a liquor store and a bar.

Being on call all the time, Cole couldn't even have a beer. He's eager to sit on a barstool again, so I tell him to go ahead without me.

I don't drink in bars anymore. I find the service too slow.

Cole leaves, and I settle in with my boxed wine and the remote control.

I can breathe again.

Leave the Water

Early the next morning, we check out of the motel, pack the car, and drive to a nearby diner. Cole and I enjoy comforting diner food, perfect for treating a hangover. We pass a plastic bag filled with aspirin over our eggs, toast, and a large plate loaded with hash browns. I keep asking the waiter for more refills, and after my third ask, he leaves the pitcher. Cole fills me in on the local characters he met at the bar last night. I feel like a dried-up sponge, and my stomach drops a few feet when I remember my promise to quit drinking. We don't mention my drinking. I want to ram the butter knife through my thick skull, but I drink more ice water to swallow the thought. I'll feel better once we get moving again, and I make a private vow never to drink again. I've never made a vow before. Maybe that'll help. I jump as the cash register drawer slams shut and a few plates crash to the floor in the kitchen. I scowl at the bright lights. I feel dizzy but smile at Cole. We get back on the road as soon as we pay the restaurant bill.

I dig around my backpack for an antacid and find the notebook I bought yesterday. I open to the first page and in small, red, handwritten letters, it says, "I can help."

I wish I'd noticed this yesterday. Why didn't I look? Why didn't I get two? Why did I drink again? Do I even have a pen?

I look around and find a pen on the floor and decide to write, "I Can Help." I write a question with my right hand and answer using my left, a technique I read in a magazine.

—⁂—

Dear I Can Help,

There's no way I can stop drinking. I've tried a thousand times.
Then consider 1,001 your lucky number. You're curious already. It'll be fun.
Fun? Are you out of your mind or just annoying?
Luckily, I am out of my mind. You could be out of your mind too. Being out of your mind is freeing.
Your cheerfulness gives me a headache. Please stop.

—⁂—

I challenge "I Can Help" with more skepticism. I keep getting jolly responses, which annoys me further. "I Can Help" insists I can quit drinking. I vigorously disagree until the road drops and the view catches my attention.

The road turns and dips through rock formations and along mesas that jut abruptly from the flat desert floor like guitar solos thrown into a Bach concerto. I feel like we're driving on another planet, and I enjoy the newness.

Our hotel for the night is on an Indian reservation. Panic floods my stomach when I remember it's a dry reservation; no alcohol allowed.

At the next gas station, I slip into the liquor store next door and buy more wine. I sneak the wine into my duffle bag while Cole buys a few hot dogs. I feel guilty and relieved. I'm so tragically predictable, like an elephant without a memory. A typical day swearing I'll never do something I inevitably end up doing.

I zip up my duffle bag and carry it through the lobby. The clerk invites us to an event in the lobby that night, and I don't meet his eyes. Cole says something I can't hear. I feel guilty about smuggling in the wine and walk over to the elevator while Cole finishes checking in.

Chapter 2

Where to Start

The following morning, Cole drives because I'm hungover once again. I wanted to get away so badly, but now that we're on the road, I'm starting to think I could have done things differently. When I begin to relax, panic jolts my heart, like invisible electrodes firing at random. I remind myself that I always feel panicky when I'm hungover. I swear I have the shortest memory on Earth. Hangovers and regrets seem like best friends, determined to reunite as often as possible. I wish I could call my mom and ask her advice. She'd make me feel better. I don't want to think about the past, but memories are difficult to keep at bay without alcohol.

During the first Gulf War, about ten years ago, I called my mom from work and couldn't reach her. This was very unusual because we talked several times a day and knew each other's schedules by heart. She lived 1,500 miles away, but our phone calls made my boring job marketing ski vacations bearable.

11

I kept calling to no avail. A clear knowing enveloped me. I wasn't hysterical, but I knew something serious had occurred. The knowing came with a clarity I'd rarely felt before.

I clocked out early, which wasn't unusual. I arrived each day at 9:00 a.m., and by 9:30, I wanted to leave. Sitting at a computer for eight hours felt so uncomfortable, like wrestling an invisible alligator. I fought each day to stay until 5:00, but by 4:00, I had to leave or risk screaming.

Once home, I opened a bottle of wine, wondering when or if I'd hear from my mom. Cole came home, and we waited together on the couch. A few glasses later, my dad called.

"Well, silly, your mother took a spill down the stairs this morning," he said without saying hello.

My mom had surgery on her back just last week. "What was she doing upstairs? Your bedroom is on the first floor."

"I don't know what she was after. You know the treads on this old house are worn down."

I braced myself. "Is she okay?"

He laughed but didn't explain why. I walked into the small kitchen, finished my glass of wine, and poured more into a tall travel mug to disguise my drink from Cole. "Well, I waited for her to come to, which took about two hours…."

"You didn't call an ambulance?" Fury and fear pounded through my head until my ears ached.

"The corpsman said it wasn't a concussion, and he stitched up the gash. It only took a few stitches."

I wanted to scream: *Why didn't you call an ambulance? or How could you possibly think being passed out for two hours meant there wasn't a concussion?* But I knew my dad. I knew if I got angry, he'd shut me down. I needed to know what happened. Instead, I swallowed more wine and asked, "She didn't see a doctor?" I walked back into the living room with the travel mug and gave Cole a look of disbelief. Cole looked concerned, and my hope waned.

"I drove her to Walter Reed, and it was pretty empty. Most of the personnel have been deployed to the Gulf. There weren't many doctors on duty."

I drew in a breath to ask another question, but he interrupted.

"—Now, don't get upset. I know how you get. The corpsman got the job done and said it didn't look like a concussion to him."

There was so much wrong here I didn't know where to start.

"Can I talk to Mom?"

"She's in bed with an ice pack on her head. She's pretty worn out, as you can imagine. She'll call you in the morning." He hung up.

My birth wasn't a celebration for my dad. My brother and sister were nearly teenagers, and he probably wasn't looking forward to having a baby in the house. My mom said his anger towards me started before my birth. He complained about me to everyone.

My mom always made things better. I couldn't consult her about her fall, and I felt lost. Cole once told me he'd known my mom grew up poor because she made the best gravy. He'd said, "Only the poorest folks know how to take leftovers and make it the best thing you've ever eaten." My mom could make almost anything better with her unique point of view or make a delicious meal with only a few meager ingredients.

Cole and I talked briefly about what had happened. I wanted to open another bottle of wine to help me not think. I hoped the wine would drown out my father's lackadaisical response to what sounded like a nasty fall, much less an injury, to the most important person on Earth.

I slipped the last wine bottle from the kitchen pantry into my backpack and told Cole I needed to work to get my mind off my mom's fall.

I shut my office door and listened to the news about the war and all the lies that made it possible. I attempted to open the second bottle quietly, but corks are loud. I didn't buy boxed wine for fear the liquor store clerks would think me an alcoholic.

I also bought a bottle of red and a bottle of white in case my "dinner guests" expressed a preference. Taste or quality didn't matter to me anymore. Wine was wine, and boxed wine would mean fewer trips to the liquor store where I'm sure I wasn't the only customer with imaginary dinner guests.

The tires rumble across gravel and I look up. Cole pulls into a gas station an hour from Phoenix. He asks if I can drive for a bit. I'm feeling better. I don't like remembering. Memories come with emotions that require wine.

Cole likes to drive the speed limit. I'm happy to speed things up a bit. According to "I Can Help" I still have a chance to put drinking behind me. But I can't help but wonder if the hotel in Phoenix has a bar.

Chapter 3

A Little Back and Forth

We arrive at our hotel in Phoenix, and we each take a duffle bag up to our room. Cole calls his sister to tell her about our trip so far, and I apologetically mouth that I forgot something in the car. Then like a bloodhound, I seek out the nearest supply of liquor.

I find the bar, but it won't open for another two hours, which feels interminable, like waiting for sand to turn to glass.

I go back to our room and change into my bathing suit and lie to Cole about going for a swim. I suspect we both know the bar sits next to the pool. Cole says he's going to take an afternoon nap. I've told him I'd quit drinking so many times I think he deals with his disappointment by sleeping. I hate that I've let him down, but I'm on a mission.

I find some mini wine bottles in the gift shop. I sit in our car and finish them off, but I'm still as sober as a crowbar.

I go back to the gift shop and ask the clerk if they have any more wine, and he says I bought them all. I'm embarrassed and annoyed. I wish I'd loaded up at a liquor store before I started drinking. Now I'm too paranoid to drive. I don't see any stores within walking distance, only office buildings.

I move the car a few parking spaces over with a view to the bar door. I'll know the second they open.

I find a pen in the center console and write "I Can Help" to pass the time. I'm not used to the desert heat and turn the air conditioning to full blast. I prop my dinosaur notebook on the steering wheel.

—⟋⟍—

Dear I Can Help,

We've not heard from the people who hired us for the job overseas. What if I made a mistake? I hate myself right now. I want a glass of wine. Or five. Or ten. What can I do? Can I still get your help?

Dear Sylvia,

I've eavesdropped on a million lives waiting for someone to ask. It's never too late.

Where are you writing me from? Personally, I think I'm nuts. Maybe delirious, too.

Feeling nuts isn't unusual in modern times. I'm from a time when humans still lived in healthy communities. Humans flourish as cooperative beings, one vital part of a worldwide ecosystem.

I lived far away, and so long ago, you'd probably think I lived in a cave.

That makes me think of prehistoric times. Are you an ancestor of mine?

In a sense, we—

You lived in a cave? Then I'll call you Cave Woman.

That's fine. What you call me doesn't matter. But please keep writing.

Sure. Whatcha got for me? Might as well write while I can. Do they let inmates in insane asylums have pens?

I know you've promised you'd stop drinking many times before. Since the alcohol isn't working, why not stop now?

A little back and forth might make the clock move faster. I'll play. I'll stop drinking if it'll help repair some hurt I've caused. At least until the bar opens. What level of difficulty are we talking about here?

Down the road, sobriety will not be as tricky as the panic and worry you're feeling now.

Down the road?

Just by asking and listening, you've already begun to mend. You'll stop and start and feel like a mess at times. Just keep asking. And breathe. Your body needs you to breathe to release tension. You have tremendous pressure restricting your breathing, which adds to your panic.

I'm afraid if I breathe and relax, a dam will break, and the flood of regrets will never end.

Many modern humans share the same worry. You have a planet filled with people bracing against feelings they believe are unbearable. It's no coincidence you also have a world filled with addictions.

I don't know if I can bear how I feel right now.

You will feel uncomfortable at times, but it's nothing you haven't felt and survived before. No feeling lasts forever. Wade in, breathe, and give your poor jaw muscles a break from all that compression.

Together we'll reach the other side. Are you willing to put your toe in the water?

If I put my toe in the water, I won't be swept away?

You won't be swept away. You only have shore to gain. Imagining the cool sweetness of water can lessen agitation.

I can't get comfortable, like my kayak got swamped, and I can't find a paddle to right myself.

I understand. We'll get you a paddle. And some kayaking skills.

And right now?

All that muscle tension and shallow breathing tells your Survival Brain you're in danger and pulls you into the Red Zone of the fight, flight, or freeze response. The Survival Brain, in turn, signals the nervous system to stay in a near-constant state of emergency.

What we'll call the 3F Red Zone.

Does 3F stands for fight, flight, or freeze?

Correct.

A little warning might be nice.

You do get a warning, what we'll call the Yellow Caution Zone. I'll help you recognize the signs of the Yellow Caution Zone so you can avoid an unnecessary fight, flight, or freeze response.

And the Survival Brain?

The Survival Brain, a short name for your entire survival system, runs all the processes in your body that keep you alive. You'll need some—

I see movement near the entrance to the bar, throw the notebook aside, and grab my backpack, only to find the bar door still locked. Are they understaffed? Should I complain to the manager? This is a reasonably large hotel; I can't be the only one waiting for them to open. Why aren't my fellow drinkers banging down the door? I go back to the car. Please, Cave Woman, help the time move quicker. I restart the car and the AC.

—⟋⟍—

Dear Cave Woman,

Where were we?

Dear Sylvia,

Helping you understand what's happening in your body. Getting you some practical information. Helping you discern a craving from a survival response.

That sounds so annoyingly reasonable. Am I mistaking a survival response for a craving?

Among other things.

I do freak out. I feel like I can't bear to feel one more thing, so I drink. But you're saying I'm in danger?

Not necessarily. You're reacting to your natural survival system as if it's the source of danger. You need the 3Fs —

Can you just get rid of my 3F Red Zone?

No, you wouldn't want that. The 3F Red Zone is only one aspect of your complex survival system. You're always using fight, flight, or freeze throughout each day, which gives you motivation, flexibility, passion, rest, liveliness, and many other things that make life interesting.

I think I bounce between flight and freeze. I wake up hungover, angry at myself, overwhelmed, and drowning in anxiety. I just want to run far away. Instead, I jump into work or cleaning or some new outlandish scheme until I collapse. Toward the end of the day, it's all I can do to get to the liquor store, get home, and guzzle wine.

That's a good example. Stick with me. You wake up from being knocked unconscious—or as you call it, passing out—and you immediately attack yourself for drinking again. Under attack,

the Survival Brain cues the nervous system to fight or flee. You work frantically all day, berating yourself the entire time. To the Survival Brain, this looks like fight or flight didn't work, so it sends you into a freeze response. That's when you collapse.

All because I beat myself up?

Your culture teaches that self-reproach motivates but berating yourself contributes to the reason you collapse or freeze.

Collapse is a good word. Toward the end of the day, I feel so depressed, like I'm walking through knee-deep tar. The decision to drink gets me moving. I get super revved up about going to the liquor store. Ironic, after a day of swearing off the drink forever.

This may seem ironic, but it makes sense. When you decide to drink, you feel relieved, as if the danger has passed, so your survival system gives you a kick of adrenaline to get you moving again.

A kick of adrenaline did propel me to the liquor store. I swear nothing could stop me. So how do I make the adrenaline kick go away?

It's a powerful kick, but not something you want to make go away. The ability to emerge quickly from a freeze response can save your life. Or prevent you from killing someone else and ending up in prison.

But if it hurls me toward drinking, what can I do?

For now—and remember we're just starting—you can cue your Survival Brain to unfreeze simply by breathing if you're not in immediate danger.

Oh geez, this breathing crap again. I've tried every breathing technique on the planet. This is rubbish.

I understand your skepticism. The breathing techniques you tried in the past aimed to get you into a meditative state.

Breathing assists the nervous system in releasing the 3F Red Zone. No enlightenment or bliss state to achieve. But if the breathing makes you feel more agitated, we'll stop right away. We'll learn many things together. If breathing doesn't ease the agitation, something will. Stay tuned.

What am I trying to achieve?

Some trust.

Not going to happen. I don't trust myself at all.

Trust, in this instance, means recognizing a survival response when you're still in the Yellow Caution Zone, which builds a sense of safety within your mind-body system.

I'll recognize what's happening and not freak out?

Precisely.

Science is relaxing.

I agree.

I find this interesting, but how does this info help a poor schlub craving a few dozen drinks?

To reserve the 3F Red Zone for when you're actually in danger instead of when the gift shop sells out of mini wine bottles.

I rarely feel safe, especially around others.

I know. You'll steer clear of danger more effectively without the constant activation in the 3F Red Zone. Asking for help will also feel less daunting and permit healthier heartfelt connections.

I only feel a heartfelt connection to Cole, and I can't follow him around all day.

No, you can't, but you can feel the connection whether you're together or not. You can feel connected to life in general, to your senses, to loved ones in this world or in mine, to that spider on the wall listening to our conversation who's

curious if you'll make a life-changing decision, to the tumbleweeds blowing by, inviting you to roll like them. At some point, addiction becomes involuntary but can be understood and resolved. Does that bring you some relief?

I'm relieved to know all this commotion inside isn't just an unstoppable craving. I get it. And I admit my jaw has loosened a bit. But there has to be more to recovery than just learning about the 3Fs.

We've talked about your Survival Brain, but we've barely touched on your Creative Genius, your diligent, helpful emotions, and your intuitive abilities. When you begin to unwind a chronic 3F Red Zone, you'll recall your ability to connect with the living world. You'll also meet the fourth member of your survival ensemble; Ease, as in fight, flight, freeze, and ease.

Ease comes with drinking.

Ease doesn't mean you won't have emotions.

Then what's the point?

You'll find out.

Oh, alright, what do I have to do?

All you need to do is not drink anymore tonight.

I'll do it. I'll quit. I won't ever drink again. But why is alcohol the only thing that quells anxiety? I just want to stop feeling so panicked all the time. Maybe I can't do this. It's complicated because—

I stop writing. My heart revs up, thudding like an avalanche in my chest. I struggle for breath, which makes my heart pound even harder.

I lean to my right and look down the hotel breezeway to see the bar is still closed. Damn, I need to drink now.

I reach behind the passenger seat and pop the lid off the cooler and find two bottles of water left from our trip. The ice cubes have melted, but the bottles still feel cool. I put one behind my neck and drink half of the other in a few gulps. My lips go numb, and I know the numbness will soon spread to my tongue and cheeks.

I pick up my pen and try to focus on the page.

———※———

Dear Cave Woman,

I think I'm having a panic attack.

Dear Sylvia,

The water will help. Now, put one hand on your heart. Can you feel your heartbeat?

Big time. Like a bass drum.

See how your upper chest moves in and out?

Yeah.

That's you hyperventilating, which only adds to the panic. Instead, keep your chest still and breathe so your lower belly pooches out.

Let my belly pooch out? Are you crazy? Is that even legal for an American woman?

If sucking in your belly is a law, I declare it null and void. Slow your breathing down. Proudly let your tummy bulge. Release your stomach muscles. You're breathing like a sewing machine and making yourself light-headed. Instead, breathe low and slow.

Exhale a bit longer than you inhale.

That does feel better. Thank you. Panic attack averted. But now I feel fat.

Doesn't feeling fat feel wonderful?

No, I meant—

I was skinny and admired the women with big bellies. Everyone did. You're lucky.

It's called a spare tire.

Then we'll call this Spare Tire Breath.

I don't think you'll get much traction with that, but it works for me. Panic attacks feel so awful. Why did I have a panic attack?

You committed to not drinking ever again. Then you started thinking about the times you failed and felt over-whelmed by looking too far into the future.

What is a panic attack, anyway?

You need to breathe out carbon dioxide, not just take in tiny sips of oxygen. The panic attack alerted you to breathe more fully. Maybe it's also time to find some help-ful humans?

Do I call 911 and say I'm having a panic attack because the bar isn't open yet and a Cave Woman is telling me I breathe wrong?

You know what I mean; asking for help with addiction.

I don't like asking for help. Can't I battle this by myself?

You don't need to do battle at all. Overcoming addiction is not a battle. Recovery is not combat. Drop that idea right now, along with those tight shoulders. You can't fight addic-tion. Fighting with yourself just ramps up the stress and sends you into the 3F Red Zone and makes you want to drink again.

I've asked for help before and felt embarrassed and awkward. I've often received the opposite of help. I hate asking for help.

Along with most of modern humanity, you learned that ask-ing for help equals admitting defeat. But admitting the truth to yourself brings great relief and lowers your stress levels.

Admitting you have a drinking habit will liberate you.

I can't even grasp that idea. I hate this. For me, drinking feels liberating. I'm so tense. I feel like I'm being crushed by an invisible boa constrictor.

Right now, you can decrease the tension a bit. Your choice, my baby boa. Breathe just a little bit slower. No need to hyperventilate.

Is this a trick to get me to relax? Because I've tried relaxation techniques and they don't work.

You're right about one thing. You can't relax away a survival response when you're in mortal danger. Attempting to relax when a lion, or a truck, is headed straight for you could prove deadly.

But breathing and moving a little will help ease a panic attack when conditions are relatively safe. You just breathed your way out of a panic attack. Give our conversations time. There's so much to talk about. So much to learn. So much self-pressure to alleviate.

But just start here: Notice the rhythm of your breathing when you feel panic rising. You were born knowing how to breathe from your diaphragm. Practice the Spare Tire Breath several times a day. Expanding your spare tire also expands your lower back and pelvic area, alleviating strain. No need to go overboard and take massive deep breaths. Pause for a second after an exhale.

And remember, you have me now, too.

Oh yeah, maybe I'm drunk after all. This is so confusing. If I don't drink enough to fall asleep, I'll be awake all night and in agony.

Initiations are necessarily difficult and, at times, agonizing. Think of recovery as a rite of passage, the initiation from child to adult that you missed by not being raised in a supportive, wise community. A healthy initiation will leave you feeling prepared for life's challenges, not lost or confused.

I went through adolescence. Wasn't that terrifying enough?

No, because you didn't have enough guidance. No one in your life did.

Can I say no to this initiation?

Of course, you get to choose.

But?

An uninitiated human is perpetually stuck in an adolescent hall of mirrors; halfway between childhood and adulthood, innocence and arrogance, dependence and freedom. Many so-called mental illnesses and addictions exist in this stuck state. In your culture, recovery from addiction has become one way to wake up from this ruinous and distorted adolescence.

Addiction has become a de facto rite of passage?

No, recovery has become a de facto rite of passage, and the initiation process forever seeks completion. A complete initiation has several phases. I'll explain each phase as we proceed. Are you ready?

Is anyone ever ready?

Good point. We've already started. Let's continue.

I hate this. I feel sick. Can we start tomorrow?

Why continue something you said wasn't working? You're pumped so full of adrenaline that more alcohol would only be like a drop in the ocean.

Let me tell you a story—

But I have so many questions.

I know, and we'll have time to discuss them all. But, right now, it'll do you good to take a break, sit back, and listen.

Let me tell you a story.

A little girl in our community wouldn't stop talking. She drove even the most patient to distraction, and we were a very patient people. We'd sent the little girl to a deaf old man, thinking her jabbering wouldn't bother him. She followed the man everywhere and wouldn't give him a moment's peace. She drove him to go fishing even though we had enough fish to last many months. We usually frowned upon fishing when we already had enough, but no one stopped him.

Her constant chattering drove him to fish the same river that left him without his hearing. He'd slipped into a churning springtime river several years prior—while fishing no less—and by the time he found his way back to us, he couldn't hear a thing. He hadn't fished since but needed to get away from the bothersome little girl.

We knew why she couldn't stop talking. We'd been remiss in sending her to him. She'd sat with a sick friend and mimicked the words she'd heard our healers say to other ill community members. She'd fallen asleep and awoke to find her friend had died. After that day, she talked incessantly, perhaps in the hopes of keeping everyone alive. Or maybe because she couldn't bear the self-blame she stacked on herself when she stopped talking.

One evening, we took her to the fire and walked with her through the bedrock of her grief. She drew her memories in the dirt until she could see why she was obsessively saving us and mistakenly blaming herself. We danced until her talking became a part of the rhythm in our hips. We sang until we attracted animals. Their eyes reflected the flames, and their understanding transformed her pain into compassion for all creatures, including herself.

—⚬—

Dear Cave Woman,

She was you, wasn't she?

How did you know? Yes, she was. I began to study with a healer in earnest after that. I'd experienced the repeating patterns your people might call obsessive-compulsive behavior or addiction. All these patterns occur when old wounds and misunderstandings get stuck in the mind-body system, unresolved and lodged tight. This story is one reason I know how to help if you'll let me.

I will, I think…maybe. I mean, yes. Thank you.

—⚬—

I put down my pen and drink the last of the water, lean against the steering wheel, and cry for the little girl who couldn't stop talking. My mouth opens to scream, but nothing comes out. I cry for a few minutes, then abruptly stop. I clean my face with a napkin I find on the floor. I take a few Spare Tire Breaths and sigh.

An orange glow surrounds me, which seems to emanate from the floorboards. I look up to see our hotel ablaze with red and orange as if the sunset broke loose, landed in the parking lot, and splashed against the sandy stucco.

I open the windows and turn off the car. The fresh breeze pushes out the stale air.

The bar opened a while ago, but I don't want to drink. Oddly, the sunset is more compelling.

Chapter 4

Ginger Gooies

I open our hotel room door, and Cole seems surprised to see me. He probably assumed I'd found the bar, but he doesn't comment. I say I'm tired and need some sleep. The room smells stale, matching the worn olive carpet, but it feels roomy for the price. I change into a cool cotton nightgown and brush my teeth. Cole and I pull off the bedspread and lay on the sheets. I flip around the channels looking for a movie to watch. I can't settle on one, but I can't stop searching either. I look over at Cole and see my monotonous channel surfing has lulled him to sleep.

Reaching over the side of the bed with one arm, I slowly and quietly drag my backpack onto my stomach. I dig around inside, put the pen in my mouth, the notebook on my chest, and a bottle of water on the nightstand.

—◈—

Dear Cave Woman,

I have a question I bet you can't answer. Why the hell am I in the extreme end of the 3Fs so often? You called it the 3F Red Zone.

I've never experienced severe trauma. I feel like I'm in the rapids without a paddle, and it makes no sense. My life hasn't been *that* hard.

You did have difficulties as a child. Your father—like all good plutocrats—delivered daily diminishments. You felt trapped and helpless, and that's traumatic. Any difficulty can cause the powerful Survival Brain to generate protective patterns, including physical effects and addiction. One tiny grain of sand can make for a very large pearl.

But millions of people have a similar upbringing or worse. Although, I'm hyper-alert an awful lot.

My senses are painfully wide open. Sounds often seem too loud. Lights feel too bright. I'm intuitive but also paranoid. I feel panicked a lot, like my kayak might tip over at any minute.

And know the Survival Brain works without you having to remain in a panic. There's no need to spin through the maelstrom of everything that could possibly go wrong when you're not in immediate danger.

I do that all the time; I try to remain aware of all the things that could possibly happen, but you're saying that knowing all the worst-case scenarios isn't helpful?

Only in small doses. The Survival Brain can run every possible danger without you deliberately searching for what could go wrong. You don't need to study worst-case scenarios.

That's why I can't sleep unless I drink. That's why I clam up a lot. I'm reviewing everything that could possibly go wrong so I don't look stupid or get blamed for something I didn't anticipate. How do I let the Survival Brain do its job?

A paddle is strapped to your kayak. Tonight, the paddle will be your pen, dig in and push off. Together, we'll navigate rough waters, pop out of whirlpools, and race down green waters.

—◊◊◊—

I put my notebook aside, sneak over to the window, and look outside. A man tries to push another man in the pool next to a table filled with drinks. They laugh, pushing and pulling against each other. Two women recline in lounge chairs, towels wrapped around their waists, sipping frozen margaritas. The idea of sneaking down to join the party feels exhilarating. I smile wickedly but then feel Cave Woman's eyes on my back. Dig in, push off, use my pen. I slump back to bed, feeling mournful like I'm missing my own birthday party.

—◊◊◊—

Dear Cave Woman,

Why does it feel impossible to stop drinking once I've started?

Alcohol is a toxin. Your liver works diligently to remove toxins as efficiently as possible. Unfortunately, alcohol leaves little room for the liver to do its usual job of processing carbohydrates, proteins, and fats, which throws off glucose and hormone production. Alcohol causes you to lose more fluids than you ingest, increases stimulants in your brain, and creates blood sugar spikes, all resulting in low quality sleep, tiredness, trembling, irritation, nausea, and sweatiness, which can feel dreadful. All these signals yell, "Stop consuming toxins!" but you, and millions around the world, drown the warning in more alcohol.

I thought the dread meant I couldn't go without alcohol. It makes sense why cravings are hard to ignore. Does my body need alcohol?

Ask it.

Body, do you need alcohol? I feel my stomach muscles recoil as if I've been punched in the gut. I'm guessing that's a no. What does it need? What can I do?

Do you have something to eat?

I have something called "Ginger Gooies" for carsickness.

That's basically candy. They'll help raise your blood sugar and ease the old habit of "fixing" these warning signs with more alcohol. Your blood sugar has been on a wild ride since you first began drinking and eating foods that quickly raise and drop your blood sugar. Eventually, we'll get that evened out, and you won't need the sugar at all.

—ᎠᏔ—

I set my notebook aside and pull the bag of Ginger Gooies from my backpack and eat a few. Then a few more. Then a few more.

—ᎠᏔ—

Dear Cave Woman,

Okay, that helps a little. But now I can't stop eating Ginger Gooies. I may eat the whole bag. I do feel calmer, less panicked. Less sweaty, too. Now keep me distracted. I'm curious, what did I miss in adolescence?

Let me talk about childhood and the Survival Brain for a minute. Through the first seven or so years of life, children slowly absorb all the knowledge they need to live successfully as healthy adults. Humans are basically in record mode during early childhood. The recording stops around the age of seven, the Survival Brain stores the recordings, and the playback begins.

Why?

Because it would be impossible to remember everything needed for safety and survival. The playback helps you avoid danger automatically.

For example?

For example, entering a canyon with low dark clouds approaching wouldn't be a moment for debate. You'd turn back without a second thought because the playback from early childhood immediately clarifies the dangers ahead.

I'm afraid to ask what my playback sounds like.

Ah, that's the question, isn't it?

Is this what's called self-talk?

It can seem like self-talk, but that's an unfortunate phrase. Especially for our work together. Self-talk implies you're at fault for the initial recording.

The playback might not favor me much. Or favor women in general. Or minorities.

In modern times, the early recording can be highly unreliable.

This makes me think about the unreliable narrator I heard about in an English class. The unreliable narrator is a character spinning a tale of lies, but you don't find out the deception until later in the book. Eventually, you'll question your earlier allegiance.

This will work brilliantly for our purposes. Unfortunately, what was once a survival mechanism, in modern times, has become an Unreliable Narrator.

I have an Unreliable Narrator in my head? This makes so much sense. I can see myself walking along with slumped shoulders as the Unreliable Narrator tells me I'm lower than dirt. That rotten scoundrel. How do we evict him?

Remember, it's a recording. Not a person or a persona. We can record over the Unreliable Narrator, bit by bit, with truer guidance.

How did your community raise children to have a healthy narrator?

By watching children have fun and play. Through a child's favorite play, the adults could see what a child might enjoy doing when they grew up. Weaving the child's preferences with our encouragement helped build self-regard and a supportive Inner Narrator. Naturally, the Inner Narrator could scare the living daylights out of you when threatened. But the fright was temporary and useful.

How did you track a child's preferences?

I'll give you an example. If a child enjoyed building little shelters and enclosures, rivulets, and dams, they'd kindly be given instruction on home building and irrigation. If a child remained engaged and began to innovate, we knew we'd found the right track for them.

Really? Your children found their path in life by playing? Oddly, that makes perfect sense. What a terrible thing to lose. I feel ripped off for all of humanity. We desperately need innovative ideas.

We enjoyed watching a child realize that what sparked their imagination could also contribute to our community. Their fascination showed an engagement with life, the very point of being on Earth. We thrive on innovation. Every healthy community does.

I can't imagine a world where people get to play and work with what fascinates them most. I wish I could live in a time like that. Most people I know hate what they do or hate working. My mom encouraged me, but my dad mostly gave orders.

Giving orders isn't conducive to finding a child's greatest gifts.

I can attest to that. I like your way better. It sounds smart.

We thought so. Imparting the basics for a well-lived life built on a solid foundation takes years.

It sounds like I might be a seven-year-old with a drinking problem.

Your seven-year-old self has unhealed wounds. Take heart. Through initiation, we'll raise you up to full-grown.

When I was seven, I followed the cats and dogs in the neighborhood, talking to them like Dr. Doolittle. I ran through the woods, trying to strike up conversations with the frogs, toads, woodpeckers, and crows. I ran wild. At some point, I stopped running wild and just ran.

A healthy, diverse community would have been helpful. What has this got to do with drinking or not drinking?

We're working with your imagination, encouraging novel thoughts, and allowing natural sensations. This will help patterns fade that you associate with a need for alcohol.

I call it the terrible thirst.

And that terrible thirst now asks: Do you still need this pattern for survival?

My brain is changing?

Absolutely. You're also learning why addiction happened, what uncovering your own preferences feels like, and how to play a new tune.

I know I'm stuck on repeat. I feel it. Can I really play a different tune? I'm not sure I can change. The urge to drink is so insistent. I feel sad for the little girl I was when the Unreliable Narrator started jabbering. I might cry. I bet she had some unique talents that probably got lost forever.

Sadness helps your body relax. Sadness enables you to release your grip on the past. Cry as often as possible. And don't worry, your unique talents got squirreled away for safekeeping. They'll emerge when the time is right.

What should I do? What should I study? Should I go back to school? Start an animal grooming business?

Like a sluggish computer, your hard drive is full. Any programs you try and open won't run optimally. We'll rewrite outdated programs, install help menus, and upgrade your graphics and soundtracks. All your senses will work in concert. Stick with me, stick with recovery. Every day you'll hear a new note, a new tune, a whole new vibration, and rhythm.

Chapter 5

Drinking Habit Anonymous

I'm still awake at midnight, and I know I won't sleep tonight. I take a shower and quietly slide back into bed beside Cole. He's snoring softly and hasn't stirred since he fell asleep. I'm wide-awake, hearing people partying in the courtyard below, ice clattering in glasses, and empty beer bottles crashing into trash cans. Even when I pull the sheet over my face, I can't get away from the smell of beer and chlorine. I hear people laughing and doing cannonballs into the pool. I wish I had an oxygen tank and an IV drip filled with cool spring water. I've lain awake a thousand times, dehydrated, demolished by regret, and determined to quit drinking. I've also failed a thousand times, and I desperately need something different. Why can't I just stop? I seem to prefer playing the fool rather than asking for help. Admitting to Cole that alcohol has me in a death grip seems more painful than continuing to drink.

I wish I could run away and leave behind the part that drinks. Oh wait, I just tried that. It didn't work.

Will he understand why I need to meet with a group of sober people? People we've ridiculed in the past. I'm not sure how to begin.

I silently ask Cave Woman to make me brave and wait for a flood of courage. Nothing happens that I can discern. I plug my earphones into my laptop and listen to news from BBC for the comfort of a steady, impassive voice. I listen for a few hours with my eyes closed but grow restless and read about addiction on my laptop. I'm too embarrassed to type the word alcoholism and quietly switch out the laptop for my notebook. The curtains are thin, and the outdoor wall sconces allow enough light to see the page.

Dear Cave Woman,

I don't think I'm an alcoholic. I know I drink too much too often, but I can stop for a few days. Usually, I drink every other evening. I've never lost a job or gotten arrested because of drinking. I'm not really an alcoholic, right?

You have a drinking habit, yes?

Yes, exactly. That's it precisely. I have a drinking habit.

The word alcoholic keeps a lot of people from getting help. I wish the word didn't carry such a stigma. Let's make this easy. An alcoholic is a person with a drinking habit. Imagine a group called Drinking Habit Anonymous. Would you go?

In a heartbeat. Drinking Habit Anonymous meetings would be so crowded they'd fill entire stadiums. I'll practice using the word alcoholic.

Before long, the stigma will fade. Attending meetings might help switch up this drinking habit.

Sylvia, alcoholic. Got it. Thank you.

My pleasure. What's next?

Why do you talk so much about the 3Fs and the Survival Brain? **Your Survival Brain was never meant to do the job of an entire protective community. Understanding will help your mind, body, and survival system work together as equals.**

In time, you'll notice the input from your Creative Genius more easily. But first we'll get practical.

Fair enough. Understanding a little about survival responses helps me feel some relief from all the self-blame. But addiction doesn't help me survive. Just the opposite.

At one point in your life, alcohol was a safe haven—a cave of sorts—and the Survival Brain repeats what kept you alive during difficult or traumatic times. Certain habits did protect you, did help you survive, but they've outlived their usefulness. Addiction isn't a choice. You didn't choose addiction. No one does.

That's right. I don't have a choice. The power of the Survival Brain means drinking is inevitable. The bar might still be open. I can—

Hang on a minute. Your survival system is just one aspect of you. You can enlist different aspects for different needs. In the years to come we'll explore them all, but for now, I'd like you to understand your Survival Brain first.

But aren't our survival needs all-powerful?

Of course, your survival needs will remain powerful without you constantly inhabiting this ancient part of yourself. This aspect of you cannot see the future based on anything other than the past. It's like leaving a young cave child in charge of your adult life.

But I feel like I need my inner cave child. She's got the fight I need to go on.

I agree, your inner cave child does fight, but some of that fight is the 3F Red Zone. She can also be emotionally intense, raw, and irritable.

And I'm guessing wanting a quick fix?

Very good. You're recognizing your addictive aspect. You need your Survival Brain and inner cave child. You just don't want to inhabit her all the time.

What else can I inhabit?

You have all sorts of aspects you move in and out of. Most everyone does.

Like what other aspects?

If you need to get something done, you can choose to be logical, hang out with me in my cave, or jet through the cosmos gathering insights from the Creative Genius. When you inhabit different parts of yourself, you think and feel differently, and the nervous system responds accordingly. This understanding will be key to shifting your perspective, adrenaline, and cortisol levels.

For example?

Suppose you're inhabiting your inner cave child while sitting down to organize all your papers. In that case, it might not get done, and the self-recrimination will be harsh.

I'm pressuring the wrong aspects of myself to complete tasks they don't understand?

Yes, well said.

This is a lot to take in.

Keep in mind you already cycle through all these aspects of yourself. We'll just keep you from getting stuck in a particular aspect that isn't helpful to your current wants and needs.

Cravings don't feel like a choice. They're brutal. I don't have a craving right this second, but I can feel it coming back, like winter. I can't keep winter at bay. I'm just one dried-up leaf waiting for the next blizzard. I want to drink just to avoid the upcoming craving.

Plus, I don't know how to jet through the cosmos to get inspired. And what the heck does the Creative Genius do?

You'll recognize your Creative Genius by flashes of helpful inspiration.

I get my best ideas in the shower. Too bad I forget them by the time I get out.

Many people get their best ideas in the shower. The Creative Genius loves when you let your mind wander. When you focus away from the millions of zinging thoughts, fully formed concepts and ideas drop into your perception.

Why in the shower?

In your daily life, you're usually worrying or in problem-solving mode, fixating on the past or the future. In the shower, you're mildly focused on the task at hand. This is what people call mindfulness, which is far simpler than you think.

Take lots of showers?

Or worry less.

I think I'll have to stick with showers for now.

You'll learn to worry less, even outside the shower. I'll teach you how.

One more question.

Go ahead.

I've heard addiction gets passed from mother to child during pregnancy. Did my mom pass addiction from our bloodline to me?

Not in the least. Good question. Your people live in a sea of addiction. Pointing the finger at one pregnant woman is like blaming your lungs for air pollution. Patriarchy loves to blame problems on those they oppress.

Tell me more about your mom.

I don't want to. I need a break.

———ɯ——

I put my notebook aside and hear the bar staff move trash bags filled with empty bottles and drag chairs along the cement floor. Since all the rooms in this four-story hotel face the court-yard, the sounds carry. People return to their rooms, talking and laughing loudly. I use the bathroom and then get more water from the fridge. I'm terribly dry and I know it's not from the desert. I may be rehydrating for the rest of my life. I wish I'd visited the bar when I had the chance. The night ahead seems long and lonely.

———ɯ——

Dear Cave Woman,

I'm back and so wide awake, I'm afraid I'll never sleep again. I try to avoid thinking about the past, which requires constant vig-ilance.

My Unreliable Narrator is having a field day telling me I'm ridiculous and worthless and why bother when I could just drink instead.

Good job on noticing it wasn't your own voice berating you. Work with me and we'll make room for a new narration. I've got you. I'm listening.

My mom finally called me two long weeks after she fell. She was in pain from the back surgery and said her head hurt, but she tried to sound chipper. I could hear the suffering in her voice, so I kept the conversation brief. I asked her what I could do, and she said, "Nothing that makes sense." She had an appointment in two weeks to get her stitches removed. Even considering the pain, she sounded confused.

She handed the phone to my dad without saying goodbye.

He said, "Your mother has an appointment in six weeks to follow up. They said she doesn't have a concussion. We don't need to see a specialist. I trust these doctors."

I pleaded, "But she didn't see a doctor. She only saw a corpsman. She's in pain and something is clearly wrong. I can tell just by our phone conversation. She said she'd see a doctor in two weeks. Not six."

"You and your mother and that long umbilical cord. Mind your own business, would you please? I'll handle things here." I felt a familiar helplessness wedge inside my throat. I needed to talk with someone other than my dad and get her help.

I called an association that specializes in brain injuries. They told me her fall required an evaluation by a neuropsychiatrist as soon as possible. I called Walter Reed and Bethesda Naval Hospital, but they didn't employ any neuropsychiatrists or any brain injury specialists.

After multiple wars, the military is now filled with head injury specialists. My mom was a few wars short of getting the help she needed.

Cave Woman?

I'm here.

I have to stop. I can't handle anymore right now. I have my doubts this will help me sleep.

I know. With all the adrenaline zipping around your body, you weren't going to sleep anyway. But we did clear out some space in your busy brain.

How?

You wrote it out.

CHAPTER 6

Bathtub Jinn

The next morning, I'm proud of myself. I stopped drinking last night before I drank enough to sleep. Cole might not recognize the accomplishment, but it feels like a victory to me.

We ate breakfast, ran a few errands, and started cleaning the car. I took a few Spare Tire Breaths when I started feeling overwhelmed. The idea of drinking popped into my head a few times. I recognized the old familiar pattern, which helped keep a full-on craving at bay. So far anyway. I decided the discomfort felt like the strain of a ship being righted. I imagined myself buoyant yet stable and felt a wobbly moment of well-being.

We treated ourselves to a movie in the afternoon. It was a cowboy movie with aliens thrown in the mix. I like unique movies that attempt something different. Our old hometown theater had rickety seats, and we enjoyed elevating our feet in cushy recliners. The surround sound left the roof my mouth vibrating.

After the movie, I went for a brief swim, and then we stuffed ourselves at a snug and spicy Caribbean restaurant. We told the owners about our trip to Haiti, and they invited our questions. We ended up talking about food. We walked away with a long list of dishes not to be missed, region by region, spice by spice.

Back in bed, Cole fell asleep in under two minutes. I envy him. To get away from the ruckus and fumes from the partying by the pool, I take two pillows into the bathroom, turn on the exhaust fan, and sit in the bathtub. One pillow cushions my back and the other supports my notebook.

—⚬⚬⚬—

Dear Cave Woman,

I started drinking around 12 years old. I was a rebellious teen-ager, as angry as a bee stuck inside a window. How did your community deal with rebellious kids?

As they reached adolescence and sought more independence, they chafed against our guidance. We allowed them time for rebellion. At least, until they became a risk to themselves and others. That's when the initiation rituals began.

How did an initiation help people who posed a danger to themselves or others?

A successful initiation helped shape a judicious and aware adult.

Why don't we have initiations anymore?

As healthy communities were largely decimated, initiations got lost. An effective rite of passage isn't easy; it wasn't meant to be. It won't be easy for you, either.

The whole world needs an initiation.

I fully agree. Initiations awaken us to a world beyond the mundane, the place where you and I are speaking now. We also become guardians for the well-being of our communities.

I'm not ready to be a guardian for anyone's well-being.

No kidding. But you're not starting from scratch either. Everyone can draw from, embody, and reignite their ancient ancestral literacy. Not understanding all the available guidance or how to access it is at the root of nearly every problem your people experience.

I don't feel any kind of ancestral connection. I'm mixed up. No wait, I know how to feel connected and it comes from a bottle. I need wine. Lots of wine. A bathtub filled with wine. I feel such a vast emptiness, like my heart slipped down the drain and left a large hole. I know how to fix that. Alcohol helps me feel a part of something bigger, even when I'm alone. Drinking feels like home and I can't imagine living without that.

At best, the sense of belonging that comes from alcohol is temporary. At worst, alcohol devours hope and will inevitably create more trouble. How about feeling at home without alcohol?

I doubt that's possible I –

Let me tell you a story about my life, a typical night with my people.

Let me tell you a story.

We gathered flowers and leaves to make a salve that relived itching. In the evening, we gathered around the pot filled with herbs and water as it steamed over hot coals. The mixture smelled sweet and proud. The fragrance brought me back to my childhood and the times a loving hand slathered salve into my skin. As those memories flooded in, my muscles melted with the sensation. I laughed as I slipped to my knees. The memories were so strong that those closest to me also picked up on the sensation and laughed with me.

We often communicate through sensation, like all ani- mals. My memory was sent and received and sent back with love. We can also do this from great distances. So can your people. The animals have never forgotten. I hope you will remember. I hope all your people will remember.

I wrapped myself in the indigo twilight and slowly filled with appreciation for another day overflowing with grace and discovery. A waterfall of moonlight pledged me to the earth, helping me feel truly at home.

The night sky readied to tell us stories as the stars appeared from horizon to horizon. I could have turned around 360 degrees and stood eye-to-eye with more stars than I remembered from the previous night. I wondered about this nearly every night. Where do all the stars come from? Were there new stars each night?

The children got to choose whether we danced or heard a story first. Since they'd been running since sunup and their bellies were full, they threw themselves - with a great deal of theatrics - on to the ground and shouted, "Story! Story! Story!"

"The bones were larger than any animal we'd ever seen," a low, awestruck voice began. "We put down all we carried and drank some water and wondered about the animal's life, we imagined what it looked like, we thought about its death. We asked the bones and saw this animal, during its lifetime, chasing and romping with brothers and sis- ters and cousins. We saw water: Waterfalls and rain. Tor- rents of rain. Swollen rivers and streams. Animals played and ran together. The bones smiled wide, remembering a joy-filled life, and drew our tears."

We sat in silence, taking in the vision of a connected life and the stories it leaves behind. We returned our gaze to the stars and waited for the next storyteller to speak. Stories contain truth. Our bodies contain truth. Stories were our teachers and how we learned and expanded beyond the limits of our daily routine. Stories are sacred.

My bladder is bursting, so I shimmy out of the tub and use the toilet. I gather up my pens and pillows and get back in bed. When I look around, I half expect to find a campfire and a few night owls tending the pot of salve.

Even asleep, Cole's nearness encourages me. I scoot under the sheets and get as close to him as possible without waking him. The hotel is quiet. It's past 2:00 a.m. and the bar closed down. I feel brave enough to search my computer for recovery support groups that meet in the morning. Afterward, I'm still not sleepy, but I think I can rest for a while.

Chapter 7

Scattershot

We shower and dress in the morning, then I announce with a shaky voice, "I have to do something different. I'm going to see if I can get help with my drinking. I'm going to one of those dumb sober meetings." I can feel myself flush like I rubbed my face in fiberglass.

"It's free," I offer for no reason.

"Good idea," Cole says softly. We both shyly look at the floor. We've never been good with touchy-feely topics.

Two simple words and I transform from a repulsive monster into a person with a common problem. I take what feels like my first deep breath in years.

"Do you need the car for anything?" I ask.

"Nah, I'll just walk around for a while."

I grab the car keys, shove my notebook in my backpack, and walk to the front door.

"Sil, wait," Cole says.

I lean my head on the door, embarrassed to look at him. I keep my eyes on the doorknob, half hoping he'll tell me not to go, that my drinking isn't that bad.

"Love you," he says.

"I love you, too," I say, disappointed he didn't tell me to stay. I leave before I change my mind.

Since we'd met, Cole and I had done fairly well avoiding heavy arguments or conversations about embarrassing problems. At least, most of the time.

The first time we'd argued, he'd fallen dead asleep sitting up on the couch. I dubbed this "Argument Narcolepsy." From then on, when we disagreed, I'd have the entire argument with myself and announce the conclusion we'd reached in my head. Sometimes Cole added a few things, but the system seemed to work. At least that's what I thought. Maybe if I hadn't assumed the embarrassment would kill us both, I could have reached out for help a long time ago.

I drive to the meeting while closely following directions on a GPS that plugs into the cigarette lighter. When I reach the parking lot, my GPS announces, "You have arrived at your destination."

"I hope not," I answer back.

I sit in the car, waiting for the meeting to start. I punch the button to roll down the windows. The dry desert breeze reminds me of the uncomfortably hot day ahead. Quails, with plumes bobbing above their heads, run scattershot around cacti and thorny bushes. I know how they feel.

This recovery group was the earliest meeting I could find, and I'm still forty minutes early. As good a place to start as any. I read online that this group doesn't ask how many days you've been sober, nor do they talk about God. Shame and embarrassment run along my forehead and drip onto my dog-eared notebook despite the arid breeze.

My ears ring and I feel like there's a gummy worm stuck in my throat. My gut rumbles. Maybe I'm coming down with something and should come back another day. I almost start the car and drive back to the hotel. I think about telling Cole I've chickened out and pull out my notebook instead. All that embarrassment for nothing.

—⟋⟍—

Dear Cave Woman,

I don't know if I can go in. Can you tell me something to help me through this?

Yes. But it's deceptively powerful.

I'll take it. Please.

When you feel stuck, ask yourself if you're feeling mad, glad, sad, or scared.

I'm terrified. Isn't that obvious? Do you want a laundry list of why I'm afraid?

No, just the opposite. I want you to ask yourself if you're feeling mad, glad, sad, or scared and simply answer the question without listing why or how or who or when. No analyzing. No conclusions.

I'm drowning in emotions. How can focusing on fear possibly help?

Emotions are a part of your intuition, and they get your attention at lightning speed, much quicker than thoughts.

This storm of distress does feel like getting hit by lightning.

I understand. Picking just one emotion from a short list and noticing where you feel it in your body helps calm the storm.

By simplifying and focusing on just one? Oddly enough, that makes sense.

Okay, so I'm afraid, and it's in my chest. It feels like ten rusty soup cans are lodged inside my ribcage.

Is the intensity mild, medium, or hot?

Hot. No doubt.

Does the fear in your chest feel bearable?

By itself, yes.

Good.

Modern people have been taught to ignore their emotions and use logic instead, which makes no sense from a survival standpoint. Thoughts are too slow, and what we often think is logical, isn't. In the maelstrom, your emotions must shout above thundering thoughts to be heard.

Got it. Emotions talk to me faster than thoughts or logic.

That's right, and since you didn't know how to interpret emotions, they've stacked up like sedimentary rock, undelivered and unacknowledged.

No wonder I feel so heavy.

Exactly. Those stacked feelings have physical consequences that affect your health, including chronic muscle tension, pain, and addictions. Or what you call the storm of distress.

And each new emotion must work harder and yell through all that rock and a raging storm?

That's it exactly.

What can I do?

Bore a hole.

What? How?

By developing your emotion sense. Ask yourself several times a day if you're feeling mad, glad, sad, or scared. Ask the question and give an answer straight away. Whatever answer comes to mind is fine. If more than one emotion comes to mind, that's fine, too. Name and feel them one at a time.

Why do I need to do this?

To keep emotions flowing so they don't stagnate and seem

exaggerated or overwhelming. **Feeling emotions is much less perplexing than running avoidable survival mechanisms all day and night.**

Maybe there's a reason we've been taught emotions are dangerous. So I have an embarrassing question: Are emotions dangerous?

Absolutely not. Emotions guard the hive. Teaching people that emotions are dangerous leaves them vulnerable.

Vulnerable because our Survival Brain thinks a piece of us is missing?

Yes, raising humans to avoid emotions creates a belief that discomfort is avoidable. You can't entirely avoid discomfort. Attempting to ignore emotions fills the hive with tension and stress, which causes all sorts of problems, including physical issues and addiction.

Okay, okay. Don't ignore emotions.

Well, would you avoid a warning from a loyal bodyguard?

I'd duck first and ask questions later.

Good. Ducking first is always wise.

If it's helpful, think of how the Survival Brain learned to protect you from "dangerous" emotions with any distraction it could find.

Pain and addiction are distractions from "dangerous" emotions?

Yes, chronic pain and chronic habits can be a form of distraction.

What else happens when we don't acknowledge our emotions?

In your world, people either throw their emotions at someone else or stuff them. Suppressed emotions block energy in the body and cause the Survival Brain to intercede on your behalf and run survival patterns.

Sounds like we're playing a game of hot potato with our feelings. We either throw them at someone or stuff 'em.

And I just ask if I'm feeling mad, glad, sad, or scared?

It sounds simple, but It's extraordinarily effective and will change habitual distraction patterns. When you feel your emotions, and they aren't hurtled or bottled up, your Survival Brain won't see them as a threat.

I feel like I'm wrapped in a wet blanket soaked in dread, making it hard to breathe.

I'm going to take a few Spare Tire Breaths.

Okay, that helped. My shoulders dropped several inches. The fear does feel less overwhelming.

Good. When you pay attention to one emotion and continue to breathe, your other emotions can settle, knowing you're listening more closely. Stress and tension will lessen.

Now that the fear feels a bit less intense, I'd like to write what about what I fear, okay?

If it helps, please take a minute to vent.

I'm afraid they'll know I'm an alcoholic, even though that's why we're all here. How absurd is that? I don't want the truth to come out. I want to lie, so I'm afraid to speak. I want to pretend I'm fine and I don't need help. Mostly, I'm afraid I'm beyond help. I've made some stupid mistakes. No one will understand. I feel sick. I want to go home.

My little flea, you're very rocky right now. You're experiencing not only the consequences of your own mistakes but also the consequences from a broken line that happened many generations ago. All that generational hurt and blame, confusion and shame, has been passed down, generation after generation, and accumulated inside you.

It stands to reason I'd be addicted. Now that I know, I don't think I need any meetings.

Nice try, my sneaky snake. Even if they don't use these exact words, the people at recovery meetings understand how the absence of a healthy community played out in their lives. You have far more in common with them than you realize. Let the part of you that longs for community take it in, and let the part of you that feels threatened run like hell when it's over. I've got your back no matter what. I'm tough. I can take any burden you carry. I can listen to anything you have to say.

Now, tell me, what helpful input does fear have for you?

My fear says to keep going. Does that make sense?

That makes sense. Fear gives you the impetus and agility to act when doing something new. Fear offers access to your intuition. You were born intuitive, not a valued skill in your family or modern culture at large. Fear focuses perception and enhances insights. When you quash fear instead of paying attention, you experience distress and miss vital warnings.

I wish I'd had you with me all through school. I worried all the time. What a difference it would have made knowing the constant fear offered insight and not just discomfort. Although it helps now, I feel clearer.

I'm going in. Cover me.

Boundary Blindness

I leave my car precisely two minutes before the meeting starts. I find the bathroom, stand in a stall, and fan my shirt to dry the sweat. I leave the bathroom right at the top of the hour.

Seven people sit in a circle and I'm disappointed. I wanted a big crowd, so I could hide in the back of the room. The room looks like a school cafeteria with brown and tan linoleum squares and a high bank of basement hopper windows. I sit in a metal folding chair and attempt an easy and causal appearance like I've attended meetings before. It probably works as well as pretending not to be drunk while hammered.

We introduce ourselves by first name only and the chairperson asks if anyone is new. I sway a little as I stare at the floor and say nothing. Why would I want to admit I'm a novice and draw attention to myself? My stomach feels like a rock tumbler and I'm sweating despite the cool air. I'm worried my stomach will suddenly decide it doesn't like tumbling gravel and I'll throw up in the center of the circle.

They read part of some lame book and talk about what they read. Something about forgiving those who forgive themselves. I must have heard wrong. That makes no sense. I try to concentrate. I look down and notice I'm wearing my winter boots. They must think I'm crazy. Forget about the damn boots and listen.

I listen more closely as people tell their stories and feel a tiny tendril of hope. I hug my backpack against my chest and sneak a few glances at the people around me. I didn't expect everyone to look so healthy. I can't believe these people drank excessively or made fools of themselves like I did. I watch the clock procrastinate on its leaden way to the top of the hour.

As one woman speaks about her wonderful sober life and how she just wants to help others in recovery, I feel a wave of annoyance so intense, I nearly storm off. Bitter words fill my mouth and I feel like spitting them out. Or kicking something. The irritation goads my legs to run. Damn their sanctimonious sobriety and reborn goodness. I'm rotten to the core, I'm not good or innocent, and I'll never be good or innocent again. I fight the memories of the ugly and stupid things I've done while under the influence. I've quit drinking a thousand times and it never lasts more than a day or two.

When the meeting ends, I wonder why I bothered. This won't work. I leave quickly, like I have an urgent appointment.

As I drive past gas stations, restaurants, and fancy motels landscaped with giant cacti, I realize I did it. I was awkward and graceless and angry, but I did it. I never have to promise myself I'll attend my first recovery meeting again. It's done.

As a reward, I stop at a mall and shop for shoes more suitable for warmer weather. The bright, clean mall smells like cinnamon rolls and scented candles. Soft music, lively colors, and luscious textures surround me like soft hugs. I know it's all sales tactics, but right now it feels like a lullaby. I buy a pair of sandals, find a bubbly fountain, and pull out my notebook.

—⟋⟍—

Dear Cave Woman,

I attended my first recovery meeting. I didn't directly ask anyone for help, but I guess it still counts. I'm relieved I went. Attending a recovery meeting would seem so simple for someone who wasn't addicted. Remaining in my seat for an hour required wading through decades of shame and regret. I felt trapped and broken. I vacillated between wanting to stay and getting the hell out of there. I'm glad I stayed...I think. I've done so many foolish things. I don't understand how sitting in a circle and listening can ever help. My thoughts feel like springs jutting through an old mattress, sharp and uncomfortable.

I feel the annoyance coming back. I'm jumpy. My heart feels cast with sharp edges. Okay, I know. Am I mad, glad, sad, or afraid? I'm mad. Why did I get so angry when that one woman spoke about helping people?

When you were humiliated by your father and had the temerity to look outraged, he'd say, "Don't give me that; I'm only trying to help." At the meeting, the woman said she just wanted to help. Your Survival Brain matched it with moments when you felt invalidated and stifled. It sent you a little "fight" to get moving. It reminded you of when your boundaries were violated. Boundary violations bring up your protective anger.

But she wasn't attacking me directly. She didn't walk up to me and shatter my boundary.

Based on your experience, anger alerted you to a possible boundary violation. You can confirm or decline anger's warning.

I'm not sure I have a boundary at all. Can we reconstruct a boundary from scratch?

We'll strengthen your boundary, which will help you set healthier limits.

What are healthy limits? I think I have boundary blindness.

I understand and we'll change that. You'll learn to move emotions so they can return to guard duty and form a more secure boundary.

I stuff my emotions.

Everyone stuffs emotions, at times.

What the heck is an emotion?

That's a big question we've already begun exploring. But here's a short explanation:

An emotion can reflect a current situation and alert you to what needs your attention. Emotions provide a buffer between you and a full-on survival response and become helpful early responders for any situation.

Or an emotion can alert you to a similar situation from your past, what you might call an emotional flashback.

At times, a decoy emotion can shield you from one that is

less socially acceptable, depending on what you were taught.

Emotions also arise as a healthy retort to the Unreliable Narrator.

Emotions make me miserable.

Emotions don't make you miserable. They animate everything in life and give you valuable information.

And an emotional flashback?

An emotional flashback asks you if an old warning is still required. If not, the old warning uncouples from the memory, leaving the memory without an emotional charge.

For example?

Remember when you had a terrible case of poison ivy as a teenager?

Yeah, my friends and I ran naked through the woods. Drinking, of course.

Later, you avoided the woods. A place you loved during childhood. Your Survival Brain kept you away until you could consciously identify a poison ivy plant. Until then, aversion helped you avoid the woods altogether.

Aversion overreacted, don't you think?

Not compared to being poisoned.

It sounds absurd. Like a game. Why can't the Survival Brain just discharge the emotion from the memory? Why do I have to stand in the middle and feel it all?

We're not robots. Patterns and emotions need our evaluative skills. An emotionally charged memory can save your life. If that memory no longer keeps you from danger, you can feel the emotion and discharge it yourself.

Why is this so arduous?

In my time, feeling an emotion—old or new—occurred all the time. You'll learn to view emotions and survival patterns

with much less agitation. Once you learn to play, you won't need to suppress feelings and old memories with alcohol.

I do cycle obsessively in thoughts and feelings, which might explain why I drank repetitively. I'm not sure. I'd like to do things differently, though. Can you help me move some of the annoyance I feel right now? Even my legs feel annoyed.

Are you mad?

Yes, I'm mad.

Give anger your pen. Turn the page and let anger write. No limits. Let me know when you're done.

———— ✹ ————

I flip my notebook over and write out my anger, starting on the last page. I hadn't realized how angry I felt. I wonder if I drank to avoid feeling all this anger.

———— ✹ ————

Dear Cave Woman,

I filled three pages with nothing but messy curse words.

How do you feel?

Like running around the mall about twelve times.

Letting anger take the pen will usually give you a burst of energy. Go. Walk. Run.

———— ✹ ————

I pack my notebook away, take my boots off, and put on my new sandals. I take Cave Woman's advice and walk briskly around the mall until I remember I'd left my boots by the fountain. When I return, my dinged-up boots are right where I'd left them. I sit down next to them, feeling foolish. Why would anyone steal snow boots in a desert?

I'm surprised how tangibly, how physically, I felt propelled by releasing a snippet of anger. This is better than espresso, with no need to offset the caffeine jitters with loads of alcohol.

I pack up and head back to the hotel. Cole sits outside our room in a turquoise metal chair. I sit in the chair next to him and notice how strong yet laid-back he looks.

"How was the meeting?" he asks.

"Embarrassing, but not terrible. Okay, I guess," I say and switch topics. "I bought some sandals in this gigantic mall. What should we do now?"

"As little as possible." He smiles and stretches his long legs.

"I need to stay busy, but you relax. I'll go for a swim."

Inside the hotel room, I'm shocked to see it's only noon. I thought it was late afternoon. I wonder if every day will feel this long.

I take a long swim, but it's only 12:30 when I settle in a lounge chair.

What the hell happened with time? I know. I can take a shower.

I go back to the room, take a shower, and get dressed.

I'm surprised again at the time. It's only 12:45.

Maybe Cave Woman is behind this.

Dear Cave Woman,

Why has time slowed down? What did you do?

It's not me; it's your perception. You're doing something new, which makes time seem slower. Repeating your old routine required very little novelty. Laying down a new track leaves you time to discover and notice.

What did you notice about your first meeting?

You'll laugh, but I had a crazy idea before the meeting this morning. I thought the only way to alleviate my nervousness was to get drunk.

You had a habitual response to a new situation. It's understandable. Alcohol caused many problems, yet your first thought is to quell the nervousness, which is precisely what you were there to address. By the way, you're not the first person who had that idea.

I get it. I do. Alcohol makes me do asinine things but also makes the consequences disappear for a little while, adding to the pile of asinine things. It's a never-ending cycle.

The sober people you met learned, through practice, to live with their past mistakes without drinking. You can, too.

I have another confession. Honestly, I don't want to quit drinking. Can you tell me how I can drink without going overboard? I'm not sure I can live without the anticipation of drinking and the relief when I finally indulge. It seems impossible to go without a quick fix.

Can you teach me how to stop after two or three drinks?

Alcohol feels like a quick fix, but it fixes nothing. Let's find you a way of living that doesn't need a fix in the first place.

You have a mighty task ahead of you, my prehistoric friend. Living in this world without a quick fix seems impossible. People can be brutal.

How about finding a way of living where you get a natural fix?

I'm skeptical. I still don't understand how sitting in a circle and talking can help.

It's far from perfect, but the people at recovery meetings have felt everything you're feeling, and that simple fact

makes them part of your new community. They know about the tricky combination of guilt, fury, and self-recrimination. They understand craving something to look forward to; that relief when you pick up the first drink. The people at these meetings have stayed sober, even while facing brutal remorse and longing.

They weren't raised in a healthy community, so they're making their own?

As best as they can, yes.

I could barely sit still at the meeting, much less speak. It feels more like the blind leading the blind. Some speakers moved me with their vulnerability, but I didn't hear any extraordinary knowledge or wisdom.

My wise community gleaned knowledge from previous generations through storytelling. Living without that seasoned guidance would be like a large cauldron of bats flying without echolocation. They'd be crashing into one another, crashing into trees and rock walls, unable to find the cave opening or return home. It takes time.

People crash into each other all the time. Literally and figuratively.

Yes, I know. Without a healthy community to raise and teach you, tragedy is inevitable. Humans need help making sense of the seemingly senseless, and they need help healing old wounds. Just the fact that these people recovered from addiction is extraordinary. They understand you better than you can imagine. You'll find guidance if you listen beyond the words.

Listening beyond words makes no sense to me.

People feel less alone when they share their stories. This creates the hive vibe that helps remedy addiction. It doesn't

matter which recovery meetings you attend. Coming together with the wish to heal makes recovery possible. If these groups stay away from ideology, your heart will resonate with stories in ways the mind alone can't comprehend.

I guess I'll have to try harder to figure this sobriety thing out.

Trying too hard can actually work against you. How about not trying so hard?

I'd enjoy not trying. Trying always seems to lead me in the opposite direction of where I plan to go.

Now that you know where you're going, you have a much better chance of getting there. Appreciating the small connection you felt is enough for today. Now go do something frivolous.

I already did. I went to a mall. We didn't have one where we lived in the frozen north. I hated going to the mall as a kid, but today I enjoyed the flat, clean floors and air conditioning. Maybe I'll go back. Or see if Cole is hungry.

Why not go outside for a walk?

I'm not the outdoorsy type.

Oh, that'll change.

I seriously doubt it.

Chapter 8

Chocolate

It's 3:00 a.m., my third night without drinking. Usually, Cole can sleep through my tossing and turning, but he wakes up worried about the job. Since we haven't heard a word from our business partners, I have a bad feeling in my stomach. We wonder out loud if our new job will actually happen, but we change the subject and talk about finding a new restaurant the next day and make ourselves hungry. Finding a place to eat beats lying in bed wishing I was passed out, so we find a Denny's. We didn't have any all-night joints back home in the frozen north.

We slide into a slick red booth. We agree to avoid any serious topics, so I put my notebook and pen on the table if I need a distraction. I attended two different sober support groups yesterday. I didn't talk at either meeting. I'm too nervous to speak up. Cole dropped me off at one meeting, which we located by the helpful column of thick cigarette smoke rising near the entrance. He waited in the car so we could eat lunch together afterward. I feel embarrassed about attending recovery meetings. I feel as shy as when we first met but with no alcohol to ease the awkwardness. I wonder if recovery will ever seem ordinary.

"I know it's 3:00 a.m., but it always feels like this at Denny's," I say.

Cole adds, "That could be their new tagline—Denny's: Where it's Always 3:00 a.m."

We laugh until I snort, which makes us laugh even harder.

We eat every bite of food, and I guzzle about a gallon of water. The waitress frowns and gives me the "I know you're hungover" look.

"I'm not hungover. This is what three days of sobriety looks like," I protest.

She smiles and says, "Oh, honey, wait and see, it gets so much better. Wait right here." She returns with chocolate ice cream topped with whipped cream.

I open my mouth to ask how she knew, but she speaks first and says, "I've been there, and chocolate made all the difference for me. If you ever want to go back to you-know-what, eat some chocolate instead. Works like a charm."

I happily do as she suggests and eat the ice cream while Cole strikes up a conversation with a gentleman at the next table. I feel like writing to Cave Woman and open my notebook.

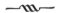

Dear Cave Woman,

I've attended several meetings in the past few days and they're helpful, but my mind still runs an endless parade of all my mistakes. How do I make it stop?

Without guidance, the Dividing Mind can run wild and spin outrageous tales.

The Dividing Mind?

The Dividing Mind quickly and efficiently categorizes our experiences as we go through each day. The Dividing Mind also generates worries about the future based on past experiences, which can seem limiting if you're not consulting with me or your Creative Genius. The Dividing Mind provides a short view, and the Creative Genius offers the long view. One gets us from point A to point B. The other provides context beyond the mundane.

Isn't the Dividing Mind the center of everything? Don't we have to judge and categorize everything?

You're always trying so hard to figure things out without inviting collaboration from your body and your intuition. Your Dividing Mind is one resource among many. It is not the center of everything; it is, however, the center of addiction.

I thought we just had to change the Survival Brain pattern and my drinking habit would disappear. Changing my entire mind seems impossible. I can't stop thinking and I can't question every thought.

You don't need to question every thought. But you don't need to believe every thought, either. A few short days ago, you believed that thinking about drinking meant drinking was inevitable.

Well, that seemed true.

But not anymore because you know that thoughts aren't always reliable.

But sometimes I randomly feel awful, like I've been struck by invisible lightning. Do I just ignore it?

No. You reassure your mind-body system that you're on the job and willing to work with sensations and feelings.

But my mind won't let my body relax. Alcohol cues my brain to relax. Without alcohol, my muscles wind tighter and tighter. What if I die from strangulation from the inside out?

Do you remember how you enjoy standing in a spring rain?

Oh, I love it when the air and rain reach the same temperature. I love pointing my face toward the sky, gathering as many drops as possible.

And your body relaxes?

It does, but it's not raining.

A few times a day or when you feel overwhelmed, imagine yourself standing in a springtime rain and help your body release some muscle contractions. Breathe in and during the exhale yield some muscle tension to gravity. Give yourself time to practice.

Cole stands up and I stop writing. I've been so busy with Cave Woman, I haven't heard a word Cole and his new friend have said.

"Are you ready to leave?" I ask.

"Wow, Sil, where have you been?" Cole asks with a grin.

"Long ago and far away, I suppose." I dare not mention Cave Woman.

"I've been talking with Michael here."

Cole gestures toward the next table and Michael, a man with long slick hair and a shabby felt hat, says, "Nice to meet you."

"It's a pleasure to meet you. Thanks for entertaining Cole. I guess I got caught up scribbling in my notebook. I didn't mean to ignore either one of you."

"I have an unusual project to build and Cole is helping me figure out how to make it work," Michael says.

"He's awfully good at that." I smile.

"It's what I like best. Are you doing okay?"

"I'm happy to scribble some more if you…" Before I finish my sentence, Cole nods yes, stands up, and slides into the neighboring booth and they both focus on the sketches Michael has spread out on the table.

I guess we're not leaving after all. I return to Cave Woman.

—m—

Dear Cave Woman,

What if I can't stop believing the Unreliable Narrator? What if inspiration has abandoned me because of my drinking?

I think you'll find our conversations contain traces of inspiration. And, one day soon you won't take the old script as seriously. You may even find some lines so outlandish you laugh out loud.

Maybe I could write the nattering down?

You already are writing down some of the nattering. Seeing your thoughts in writing helps. If you entered an Olympic event for scary thought output, you'd make the team.

I wouldn't just make the team; I'd win the gold. I can't imagine laughing at my scary thoughts. They all seem so real. The nattering keeps me down and out. Maybe it's better that way. When I dream big, I get knocked down. Every damn time.

Getting knocked down isn't your concern. Stay on the ground if you like. Rest until you feel restored. Then, you choose when and how to get up. Therein lies your power.

I get to decide? Me?

Absolutely. That's how you move forward in recovery. Even if specific ideas and dreams don't come to fruition, your imagination will be in better shape for the next new adventure.

My imagination can get pretty dark.

That's not a bad thing. I'll reintroduce you to the sensual and sanguine side of your imagination. I'll help you move more naturally with the highs and lows you experience.

What does sanguine mean?

Hopeful.

Where do I start?

Start with daydreaming. Spend time watching the stars, looking out the window, enjoying the devilish rebellion of doing nothing. It's a very radical thing to do in a mechanized world which encourages endless toil.

That sounds downright seditious.

Daydreaming exercises your imagination. Start with scribbled ideas on scraps of paper, input from—

The sunrise peeks over the horizon and blocks the view of my page. I feel alert and ready for the day ahead despite getting no sleep at all. I put away my notebook. I tell Cole that I'm ready to leave when he is. I use the bathroom and wait by the cash register. Ten minutes later, Cole says goodbye to his new friend, and we walk to the car.

In the parking lot, I ask if Cole would mind dropping me off at a meeting while he helps a family at our hotel move to their new house. I'll go to several meetings today and eat lunch with a few women also in recovery. I hope this plan will help the day go faster.

Each newly sober day goes so damn slow.

A Few Repairs

I remained pretty quiet at lunch today, but I did speak up a few times. Afterward, I felt empty but not drained. I mostly listened and accepted my role as a sobriety novice.

Cole and I decide to skip dinner and grab chips and candy from the vending machine. I get several bottles of water and fill up the ice bucket.

Cole falls asleep and I'm sitting up next to him in bed surrounded by everything I need for the night. I drink some icy cold water and start writing.

—ᴧᴧ—

Dear Cave Woman,

Where did we leave off?
In your imagination.
How about I imagine myself at the beach?

—ᴧᴧ—

I put down my pen and close my eyes and see something like television static. That can't be good. It didn't work. My heart speeds up. My body flushes with failure. Sweat beads across my face and chest. I leave the bed and turn up the AC. I'm panicked and I feel a sugar crash bearing down on me. Why didn't I eat something besides junk food? I wonder if a craving for alcohol is next.

—ᴧᴧ—

Dear Cave Woman,

I broke my imagination. I couldn't even visualize myself at the beach. I hate myself. I wish I was passed out right now. Why did we leave home in the first place? What the hell are we doing? I'm afraid I'll sneak down to the bar. I'm not in the present moment. Isn't the present moment where I can feel all blissed out and Zen-like?
Not if you're focused on the business of the Survival Brain, running worst-case scenarios about the past and lamenting the future.
Notice how your mind paints the future with a broad brush and bleak colors.
This is how I think all the time. I'm hopeless.

It may seem odd, but we're building up your capacity for loftier, more custom-tailored dreams.

Practicing using your imagination helps you build hope, which will support your recovery.

Your imagination is the playground where you'll reengage your intuition and make it possible to live more comfortably in your body, which is always in the present moment.

I'm stuck in a downward spiral.

But you noticed you're in a downward spiral. Now notice what you're making it mean.

I do spin in my mind a lot. I can daydream a bit, but I bounce right back into beating myself senseless. I've seen and done some crazy things and drinking made everything worse. How could I feel anything but awful?

Let's not go too far afield into the past or the future. Right now, I'm so glad you can see how you fall back into verbally abusing yourself. Mostly, you need to feel awful because you do feel awful. Fighting the awfulness feels even worse.

I don't deserve to feel better. I feel okay and then I feel bad for feeling okay. It's like I'm dueling with a dragon. I can't win. No sword. No training. No armor.

That's right, you don't have any training and you're saddled with perfectionism. Let the dragon do what it does. Maybe it will gobble you up or maybe it'll curl up next to you. The dragon is much stronger than you. Fighting it is futile. Feeling awful won't kill you. The dragon won't physically kill you. Feel it, and notice your mind spinning. Once you release the battle, you'll know you can survive this hardship as well. You may need this dragon energy at some point like you need all your inner hive members.

Even the emotions that feel awful?

Of course, feeling awful gives you guidance. Who or what

do you need to avoid? Can you make a change? Can you discharge some energy?

Let yourself feel awful. Practice. These awful feelings will guide you in the future but feel it first.

How can feeling this awful guide me?

When you think about pursuing an idea or a friendship and you get this awful feeling, you'll know to steer clear. That awful feeling is filled with useful information. Emotions don't make a circumstance awful. Emotions give you guidance about a circumstance. Work with your emotions and you'll reserve the 3F Red Zone for truly dangerous situations.

I don't want this awful feeling any longer. I could run down to the bar and drink it away.

Without alcohol, feeling awful will come and go. Let it. If you did something awful and didn't feel bad, you'd wonder what happened to your moral compass.

I have a moral compass? All that alcohol didn't dissolve it?

Your moral compass is a bit damaged but can be repaired. At times, feeling awful will remind you when you've run afoul of what you value most.

I have values?

You wouldn't feel so rotten if you didn't. Living from your values will come naturally once we uncover the values that get your hive buzzing, like putting on your first pair of glasses.

And lay off the sugar and junk food. Tomorrow buy some ginger without any sugar to help with nausea. Similar to a hangover, you feel intense distress during a sugar crash.

—◊—

I put my notebook aside, plug my earphones into my laptop, and listen to a woman speak online about getting sober. I'm not sure how she can make jokes about addiction but I'm actually smiling. I forget myself and my nattering mind for a time.

What a gift.

Desert Garden

After a morning meeting, I find a juice place with fresh ginger shots. I feel the nausea intensely today. As I sit in my car, I clench my jaw to keep from getting sick. Twenty minutes after the first ginger shot, I feel well enough to go back in the juice place and eat a small salad. I order three more ginger shots to go. Four days in, and I'm already eating healthy food. My drinking buddies would be horrified.

Cole calls and asks if I can pick him up. The dishwasher where he helped the family move isn't working. He may need to go to the store and get a part. I'm happy for the distraction. We get back to the hotel around 5:00 p.m.

When we first checked in at the front office, the clerk gave us complimentary tickets for the desert botanical gardens. I think we'll use them tonight. That should eat through most of the evening. Then I can swim before I slide into bed and have, fingers crossed, one more day sober.

Having plans and staying busy helped the day move at a swifter pace. We arrive at the desert botanical gardens at dusk and hear live flamenco music radiating from the amphitheater. The sky in the west looks like a hand-embroidered Mexican skirt stitched in red and yellow on a lucid blue background. Hundreds of varieties of cacti surround us, each with a distinctive charm, standing confidently. As we walk, we're serenaded by flamenco guitar and tear-stained singing only a broken heart could recognize.

I ask Cole, "Did sobriety kill me and I'm in heaven?"

"Not yet. Do you want to go listen in the amphitheater?"

"No, I'll just sit out here and scribble some notes. You go ahead."

I find a cement bench with a slanted back to lean against. I share this spot with Cave Woman and ask if she can quiet my mind. It's still in charge.

—–ɯ–—

Dear Cave Woman,

I couldn't have scripted a more stunning evening. But here I sit feeling miserable. My stomach feels nervous and is doing barrel rolls, flown by thoughts about how I'll never stay sober. How do I calm down? My head spins and spins.

You're doing it now. You're taking it all in; the birds, the sunset, the miracle of nature endlessly flaunting its prized diversity. You're also noticing what's happening inside and asking for assistance. Opening your perception in this place will infuse your senses and let your busy mind take a break. Let your senses take in this night.

What about the times when I don't stumble into a miracle for the senses?

Humming or singing a little will help set this memory. Use the memory later like medicine to quell the turmoil inside and provide your mind and body with a counterbalance. Make a list brimming with sensory-filled memories for use when you feel overwhelmed. Someday, I'll teach you an abbreviated emotion counterbalancing skill.

Oh, and breathe into your spare tire and release a bit of muscle tension into the desert floor.

Are you mad, glad, sad, or scared?

I'm sad. My heart feels like a bruised banana rolling around in the back of an old pick-up truck.

Let the music carry your heart and ask the zebra-tailed lizards, the black-chinned hummingbirds, and the thousands of butterflies to tell you what they know.

They know love without limits. Their minds feel free. They're emotional geniuses.

See? Even a bruised heart can listen.

Animals would not trade a single human possession for unconditional love and a free-flowing existence. Animals can feel the magic and awe modern humans lost long ago. They're willing to teach if you're willing to listen.

I feel like Humpty Dumpty. I don't know if all my pieces can be put back together again. Sometimes I fear I'll drown in shame and anguish.

Notice the different emotions you can evoke by imagining all sorts of scenarios.

Notice how you change the tune by altering what you imagine.

All I imagine are scenarios where I wish I'd done things differently.

How about we find a bit of neutrality somewhere in your body and help counterbalance the anguish? Your own neutral territory.

Nothing can make my disaster area of a body untroubled ever again.

What do you have to lose?

Whatever.

We'll play a game called Simply Sensational.

Seriously?

I made up the name. Just play along because in a minute you won't have a lick of attitude left.

Yeah right.

Now, you have some sensation in your lower legs. Describe it.

Okay, my legs feel mad.

Now Simply Sensational. Describe your lower legs with sensation words only.

Frustrated and—

That's a feeling.

I could ram my legs straight through the sidewalk.

That's a thought.

Churning?

Okay good. What else?

Fluttery. Wavy. Airy. When I focus on the physical sensations alone, the terrible feeling fades. This is amazing. My legs are suddenly neutral. They're neutral. How did that happen?

Isn't it sensational?

I like this, I do. Okay, moving to my knees. I definitely feel pressure in the right knee. It's growing as I concentrate. Pressure, pressure, pain. But suddenly the pain releases and now I feel a denseness, a heaviness. It changes as I pay attention. My hips feel squeezed like they're in a vice.

That's a simile. *Remember* Simply Sensational. Use only words that describe the physical sensation as closely as possible.

My hips feel achy and dry. My pelvic muscles feel tense.

Use a word that isn't synonymous with an emotional state. Maybe dense or tight.

Whatever fits best.

Oh, I see. Okay, tight. Squeezed.

Good. Keep going.

Warm but also strong. Hey, my pelvic floor muscles released a little. Still tight but less so. I'm not finding fault or finding something new—or old—to remedy. Without judgment, there's nothing in my body to fix, only sensations to notice.

Sensational. How about your stomach? You said your stomach felt nervous.

Yes, nervous. My stomach feels twitchy. Let's see what else. Also, some nausea. That's it? All that angst and worry and I can only find twitchy and a little nausea? I feel better than I have in ages.

Simply Sensational?

Effervescent.

Agreed. Effervescent.

—⁓—

I sit straighter. I look around and absorb this evening with all my senses. I feel as light and as loose as the lunar moth slowly fanning its wings on the lamppost beside me. For a moment, the eggplant sky, the emerging bats, the lizards and cacti, and the roiling flamenco taps, all feel alive inside my cells. The desert animals pause and hear my heartbeat. I almost comprehend a secret and then it's gone. I want more. That I know. Wanting more is what every addict knows intimately. I hope, for once, this longing is different.

Cole sits beside me and kisses the side of my face near my ear.

"What did I do to deserve that?" I ask as I lean into him.

"You look sweet. Livelier somehow. I just wanted a taste."

Raving Lunatic

The day after we visited the botanical gardens, I arrive a few minutes early for a noon meeting. The empty parking lot looks stark and frightening, not even a tumbleweed to fill the hollowness. I sit in my car and stare. I wonder if everyone saw me coming and decided not to show up. My stomach does a backflip. They must have called each other to avoid me.

I look at the clock and grab the meeting list from the passenger seat. I'm an hour early. The meeting doesn't start until 1:00. What a relief. I can't believe I thought an entire group of recovering alcoholics was hiding from me. I think I may have some abandonment issues left over from childhood.

—∭—

Dear Cave Woman,

I'm a raving lunatic. I don't think I'm good enough for recovery. They're going to kick me out. I have so many issues on so many levels. I'm a paranoid mess.

You're in the mess, which is perfectly normal at this stage in recovery. You noticed your inaccurate thinking. That's a sign of healing. You felt the fear and saw it as an echo from the past. Commend your fear.

Why all the fear if I'm healing?

Fear persists as a reminder to pay attention. Losing connection could prove deadly.

Deadly?

My community shared the same fear; the fear of separation or banishment. We wouldn't have survived without each other. For us, being lost or banished meant certain death. Fear of banishment is natural and a gift that reminded us to reconnect. As we unwind each emotion, you'll gain more clarity.

I'm not banished from recovery?

You assumed the worst and that reminded you of past loss and rejection.

I abandoned someone I love. I really am the worst person in the world. The panic hits randomly and clubs me over the head. Sorry about the club reference. I don't mean to offend cave people.

Listen sweet sister, this isn't *The Flintstones*. You wouldn't be alive if my contemporaries had walked around bashing each other over the head with clubs or dragged women by their hair. That sounds more like your world than mine. You think my time was uncivilized, but I see your world as far more barbarous.

I'm sorry. Our history books portray ancient times as barbaric. I'm happy to set straight any misconceptions.

As modern people separated from healthy communities, brutality spread. A few untethered humans formed new healthy communities but most formed groups that wove brutality into what you ironically now call civilization.

We are brutal. We do pretend to be civilized. I feel hopeless for the future of humanity. My heart feels like a wet box of matches. What can I do?

Right now, you can focus on recovery.

Take some Spare Tire Breaths, okay? Let's discuss this after the meeting. I think it's starting.

Okay, yes. Later.

—◊◊◊—

I sit at a large conference table in a recovery meeting at a newly built church. Black acoustic ceiling tiles dull the idle chatter to a velvety hum. This church feels fancier than the other meeting places, with plush cream carpet and linen wallpaper. Despite the posh digs, there's a respectable variety of humans represented. Confident that once I start talking, the words will flow easily, I decide to share.

I introduce myself and say, "I did something horrible to someone I love and won't ever be able to make it right—" My words halt abruptly. My mind goes blank. We sit in a painful expanding silence. My cheeks glow until the heat sears like a sunburn. I'm horrified and look down at the new-smelling carpet and mumble an apology. I put my hand over my heart to keep it from cantering away from my ribcage.

The man beside me takes the pressure off by thanking me and taking his turn to speak. "I came to the USA to open a branch of our family business," he explains in a melodic Italian accent. Once he arrived, business was endless. He felt tremendous pressure to work all the time, convinced his life depended on succeeding. At lunch with a colleague one day, he mentioned how rundown he felt, and the friend offered him some speed. The friend also gave him a doctor's name who would prescribe anything he wanted. "With wealth comes a few disadvantages. Lots of money earned me an unlimited prescription pad, and I was addicted in no time. I started drinking at night to get a few hours of sleep. Then I was, how do you say, off to the races?"

His intelligent caramel-colored eyes look squarely into each person's face as he continues his story, "One month after I was arrested for a DUI, my father died of a heart attack. He was at age sixty-two. His death is my doing. I know this. My mother tells me my sister is rarely home and I suspect she is drinking and drugging too and it's—" He chokes back tears and can't finish his sentence, but people nod their heads in understanding. He crosses his arms in silence.

After a few moments, he continues, "I used to hate when people in meetings said they are a 'grateful alcoholic.' I could not imagine how anyone could be grateful to be an alcoholic. But I may be understanding a little now. I rent a room from a fellow recovering alcoholic. I have little money. My family will have nothing to do with me.

At least, not right now. I work at a dry cleaner. The crazy part is I love this job. I have never loved work before. I love making people smile who might not smile all day. I love talking to people. They are so precious and so sad and so hurt and so full of love with no one to share with. Before, I only felt tired and a disappointment to my family. Some days I ease someone's heartache and for that I am a grateful recovering alcoholic."

He clears his throat and continues, "This is not a contest to see who did the most hurt because..." he smiles slyly and continues, "I would win." Everyone laughs and many wipe tears from their eyes, including me.

He smiles boyishly. For a flash, his burden lifts and I notice he's an attractive young man.

"I'm kidding. You know this. In addition, the pain of hurting those we love is the same for each person here. There's no difference. We come here broken and in pain but stay with the hope we can make amends. Even when it seems too late or impossible, at least in this lifetime, we must continue."

Another man speaks. Tattoos cover his muscular arms, disappear behind his T-shirt and leather vest, and reappear at his neck. He wears chaps, jeans, and large black boots. He completes his biker look with a ponytail and a long grey beard.

"I hate to make this about me, but I think I might win the contest of who hurt people the most. I don't tell my story often. Maybe once a year. But I can see the wild look in a few newcomers' eyes today and I know that look doesn't lead to anything good. I need to do as much good as humanly possible, even when it's heavy, because I killed someone.

"I did my time in the penitentiary. Supposedly I paid my debt to society. As you can imagine, there's no way in hell I can ever make up for taking a mother away from her children or a wife away from her husband. She had two sisters and a mom and dad.

"I didn't understand what I'd done until her family testified about the impact my actions had on their lives. I woke up that day in the courtroom. I was angry most of my life and suddenly all that anger and all that feeling sorry for myself was gone.

"I wanted to die, and I vowed to kill myself as soon as I could. But the judge seemed to read my mind and told me suicide was a chicken-shit way out. She said I had to do what good I could to put back some of what I took away.

"I didn't join a gang in prison. Instead, I found a mentor who helped me recognize the traumas from my childhood and taught me how to devote my life to helping others get sober. I mentor people every day and hope the woman I killed on that terrible day when I chose to drive drunk can see that our lives colliding so tragically has saved a few lives, too.

"I ask my higher power to help me do good about twenty times a day and about twice that at night. I write to the family of the woman I killed. I tell them about some of the successes I've had helping others. I tell them I make every day a mission to do good. I got a postcard back once. It said they were not surprised because she always inspired people to do good for others. They didn't want to meet me except when one grandson got in trouble with drinking and wrote me a letter. He said he felt could talk to me. Now we meet and go to meetings together. I love him like a son and would do anything in the world for that kid. We have a sad bond, but it's still a bond and a strong one at that."

The room remained silent. It wasn't an awkward silence, but one filled with a sorrowful appreciation.

Bare Mollusk

It's 3:33 a.m. The hotel is quiet but too bright. I wish I could take a BB gun and shoot out each light in the courtyard. One week sober and I haven't slept at all. I sit up in bed and then lie down again. I sigh and flop back against my pillow, hoping I'll wake up Cole for some company. I see his eyes dancing back and forth in dream mode. I wish I was dreaming. Insomnia feels like a curse. I'm wide awake and I have a question for Cave Woman.

Dear Cave Woman,

Can I have my brain removed?

Very funny. We can't remove your brain, but we can train it to engage in different activities. You need your dividing, categorizing, get-things-done mind to put ideas into action. Making a significant change is like finding first gear when you've spent years stuck in reverse. Writing helps you shift out of reverse without old patterns taking hold again.

Recovery is a bumpy ride. I can't seem to remember the things you tell me for long.

Right now, you're between active addiction and a solid recovery. You're in the bare mollusk phase. You've outgrown the old shell, where addiction provided you with an antidote against pain or discomfort. You haven't yet crafted a new shell. It's a vulnerable time.

I think recovery is killing me.

Recovery is a death of sorts. You don't yet trust yourself, and you need time to grieve.

I knew this felt familiar. Oh, blasted grief. Grieving alcohol seems weird but also makes perfect sense.

People in recovery grieve alcohol almost like they grieve a loved one.

I know that alcohol can stem the tide of grieving a tiny bit, but it'll eventually throw me in the deep end. Can we skip the grief and maybe hurry things along?

We'll go slow and take a tiered approach, so you can gain some trust and resilience.

Why? Why can't you just tell me everything right now?

Going too quickly can be counterproductive. I'll have you practice skills and review concepts in the most beneficial order. We first need to diffuse some misunderstandings that send your Survival Brain into overdrive and cause your nervous system to take protective measures, or what you might mistakenly think of as procrastination, self-sabotage, or mental health issues.

Are you saying I'm hysterical? Why? Women have been called hysterical for decades just for having an emotion. I thought you wanted me to feel emotions and now, I'm suddenly having a nervous breakdown? Wait, what did you say?

I'm saying recovery takes time.

But I want—

I know what you want. You want a life filled with camaraderie, justice, and fairness. You want to see the grander scheme. Yes?

Yes, I guess. It's embarrassing to want so much for myself and for the world when all I can do is spin in reverse and think about drinking.

Let the waves of sensation crest and fall. Everything in nature ebbs and flows, from tides to childbirth. Every thought and emotion ebbs and flows.

Now I feel embarrassed and hit by another wave of shame. Please help me.

Even when you're embarrassed, a part of your body remains neutral. Remember your little bit of neutral territory. It might be your right thumb or your left shin. Take a breather and focus on a neutral spot before you return to where you feel discomfort or intense emotion. Going back and forth between the discomfort and an area of neutrality will ease the intensity.

My mind won't stop obsessing about all the stupid things I've said and done. My mind says alcohol can ease everything. It's very persuasive. Please make it stop.

When you're overwhelmed and only living from the neck up, you're giving your Dividing Mind the job of dealing with your emotions. That's not its job. Your Dividing Mind compiles data for comparison. The Dividing Mind will take an emotion, like shame, analyze it, and submerge you in every instance when you felt shame. That's when you—understandably— sought relief through drinking.

How can I stop my mind from rubbing my face in all the times I felt shame?

Don't ask your Dividing Mind to analyze emotions. Ask your body. Where do you feel the shame in your body? The body feels and processes emotions; that's its job. Emotions make themselves known in the body through physical sensation. As you consult with your body, you'll feel more relaxed.

Is this shame an emotional flashback?

Shame, for you, often shows itself as an emotional flash-back. Addiction compounded unresolved shame. If the shame you feel doesn't dissipate soon, we'll discuss "decoy shame."

If that's true, I'll never recover. I turned beet red getting ready for school as a kid. The supply of shame feels endless. I'll be in an emotional flashback forever.

Merely realizing you're in an emotional flashback should reduce the overwhelm. You're clearing some energy.

All that alcohol didn't disinfect my energy?

No, addiction stops the flow of energy like old logs, sticks, and dead leaves clog a stream in winter. In the spring, the torrent of freshly melted snow clears the stuck debris. You're learning to disperse emotional buildup instead of clogging it with alcohol.

I need a blowout?

As odd as it sounds, you do. You can clear old hurts and traumas.

How?

Each day you stay sober clears more debris. Right now, use your breath. What emotion are you feeling?

Now I feel mad. I'm angry no one taught me I could feel emotions instead of drinking. I'm so furious.

Let's set off a volcano. Breathe into your spare tire, and before you exhale tighten your throat a bit so the exhale sounds like steam escaping a magma chamber. Feel the fear physically and let it erupt through your breath.

Oh, I like this. Let me go in the bathroom so I don't wake Cole.

I turn on the bathroom fan, sit on a towel I spread across the floor, setting my notebook aside. Volcano Breath sounds just like my anger feels. I feel like a movie monster come to life. I'm powerful and focused.

Dear Cave Woman,

Volcano Breath is visceral. The anger felt hot in my stomach and chest. As I breathed, the heat expanded beyond my skin and I broke out in a sweat. The heat dissipated like a burst soap bubble. I felt more anger in my stomach and breathed into it again, helping the fury expand and dissipate. Now, I feel clear and strong. This is amazing. Why didn't you teach me this first thing?

Lean close and listen. Your overactive mind produced a lot of worry, but the fear that grants you access to your intuition remains as clear as a birdcall.

You don't need to suffer to gain emotional insight.

I hate to admit this, but the only way I know to make things better is to suffer. Maybe If I pay a high enough price, I can buy some forgiveness.

If suffering made things better, your world would be a paradise. Suffering to atone for past wrongs victimizes you further, does nothing to help those you've hurt, and only adds to the tremendous amount of addiction buzzing through the world.

I can keep my mind?

You don't need to fire your mind. Just give it some friends to play with.

I get back in bed. Turns out there's a whole online world made for insomniacs. I listen to a jungle rainstorm and a story by a gentleman from Ireland about how he stayed sober for thirty years. Thirty years seems impossible. I also read an article saying the human body can survive with very little sleep and another one saying the opposite.

Healing Trauma

Live or die, I'm still awake as the sun lightens the courtyard. I feel stalked by a hulking impatience. Will I ever sleep without getting drunk first? I sit on the couch and crumble some peanut butter crackers into a take-out box with leftover garlic broccoli. We'd eaten the rice, but this doesn't taste too bad.

—∞—

Dear Cave Woman,

Is my initiation complete?

Now you're making me laugh. No, not yet. You have many passageways left to navigate.

About how many?

As many as it takes. Initiations are different for everyone, but I can tell you about the three stages.

Okay. What's first?

The first stage involves losing the familiar.

For me, that was quitting drinking?

Yes, or you may experience a difficult loss, an abandonment, or a betrayal.

And the second?

The second stage is an encounter with death. To you, the remote territory of recovery is terrifying, and you wonder if it might kill you.

I do. I'm afraid I might die. I've heard of people going cold turkey and it killed them. I swear, I feel like I might fall over dead at any moment. But I'm not going to a doctor. I'm afraid a doctor might laugh at me and kick me off the insurance I have back in the frozen north.

You really could benefit from seeing a doctor. Ask for a recommendation at a meeting. Believe me, many people in the medical field understand addiction all too well.

What's the third stage?

A full-blown jubilant homecoming from your ordeal as a fully engaged member of your community. This stage completes the ritual and heals trauma.

How so?

All your life you've bounced between stages one and two. You'd suffer a loss and then you abandon people or cities or entire states.

I ran away.

You felt you wouldn't survive if you didn't run.

The flight response?

Correct. It saved you as a child but that same pattern continued.

But I stayed alive.

Miraculously, you did survive. But instead of completing the ritual by declaring yourself home in the world, you'd run again. Once you stop running and complete stage three, your perspective will broaden.

Let me tell you a story.

I once threw a baby in a river. I'd recently been moved from my childhood home, filled with the adults and other children I'd lived with all my life. We usually hung out with the rest of the community but at night, in one large room with sleeping platforms at varying heights and openings for stargazing, we reveled in each other's company. Or, at least that's what I thought.

A newborn had recently arrived. Shortly after and with little fanfare, two adults escorted me through narrow stone walls. I followed, tracing with my finger the bird and snake carvings along the sandy wall. They led me up several smooth rock steps to a large sleeping room and left me there. They told me not to leave. Nothing like this had ever happened to me before or to anyone I knew.

I felt terrified and hurt. Slowly people arrived. Of course, I recognized them all, but no one offered me an explanation or looked directly into my eyes. As people readied themselves for sleep, an adult steered me toward a small empty spot and told me to lie down. Maybe, I thought, once the storytelling began, I'd be given an explanation. But soon, everyone fell asleep.

I didn't sleep, worrying about what I'd done wrong. I wondered if they were going to banish me to the wilderness and leave me to die. I'd never felt such terror.

The next day, my questions were met with laughter or silence. Something wasn't right and I panicked. I made my way to my childhood home and found the new baby sleeping. I finally understood. There wasn't room for me anymore since the baby arrived. I looked around and didn't see any adults nearby. The anger balled up in my chest and shot through my arms and I grabbed the baby, walked the rocky path toward the river, and threw him in.

Since each adult is considered the parent of each child, everyone nearby jumped in after the baby. I didn't care. I hoped they all drowned.

When they finished soothing the shocked baby, the attention chillingly turned toward me.

I thought if I lived, I'd be apologizing for the rest of my life.

"I know what happened here," said one of my former house parents, "we forgot to help her through her move."

Their voices rose with a hundred apologies as they approached. Here they were apologizing to me!

"We were sad you were leaving your childhood home to begin your initiation into womanhood. We didn't take the time to explain to avoid our own sadness. We are sorry."

"We pretended we were polite by not mentioning your move, where you would be taught by wise women to become a wise woman yourself. We avoided feeling awkward. We were wrong and insensitive. We are sorry."

"We forgot to help you grieve your childhood and begin to embrace your womanhood. We are sorry."

"We forgot to help you anticipate the wisdom and mysteries you will uncover. We are sorry."

"We spared our own hearts and trampled on yours. We are sorry."

"We love the child you are and already love the woman you will be. We didn't want you to go and we didn't want to hold you back. We are sorry."

I walked over to the baby, who had fallen asleep. I reached for him and no one stopped me. I lifted him into my arms and whispered, "We are sorry."

I hadn't acted alone. We each bore a responsibility and we would heal together.

Those who knew me best had seen me at my worst, yet still loved me. I knew I would feel this love forever.

As the baby grew, I paid him extra attention to help resolve any signs of lasting trauma. I owed him what had briefly been denied me: The full love and healing attention each human needs.

Cave Woman?
Yes?
I'm sorry.
I know.

Chapter 9

Write the Scene

I head out early to a mid-morning meeting. Afterward, I pull my car underneath a shade tree and point the air conditioning directly toward my face. Hearing people in recovery speak candidly feels heartbreaking and helpful at the same time. When I attempt to talk, I get tongue-tied. I can't write. I'm tongue-tied on paper too. Not speaking clearly worries me. Maybe addiction robbed me, and I'll never speak clearly again.

I get out my pen and notebook, but I just sit there and stare at the blank page.

I head back to the hotel but feel restless, so I find a women's meeting I can attend this evening. Cole and I eat an early dinner at a restaurant in downtown Scottsdale. I order a big salad with the best ranch salad dressing I've ever had. I ask the waiter if they have it for sale, but he laughs and says, "Everyone asks that."

We walk around and stumble onto a large library. We go inside and I take in the familiar woodsy smell of softly decaying books. I haven't seen this many books in years. My heartbeat picks up with happiness. I vow to return with my notebook.

Cole drops me off at the women's meeting and affably picks me up when it's over.

Back at the hotel, Cole asks, "Want to sit by the pool?"

I look at the bar and think, no way. But what if he's disappointed or resents me for saying no? What if my recovery will mean he's bored all the time? I take a chance and say, "I don't think sitting by the bar is the best idea right now. Is that okay?"

"Sure, it's okay. Just thought I'd ask," he says with a shrug.

I decide to believe him.

We head upstairs and watch a funny movie about a serious topic. We used to laugh more and talk after the show. We vow to lighten up and recoup our funny bones.

In bed, I ask Cole to hold me. He wakes up a few minutes later and apologizes for falling asleep. I didn't mind at all and tell him I'm fine.

Wide awake, I scooch over and pull out my notebook.

Dear Cave Woman,

My mind won't let me sleep. We haven't heard a word about the job. I left behind a family member to do this and I'm worried it might not happen.

I feel like a pool of gasoline near a lit candle. Some boxed wine would douse the flame in no time.

First, let's—

I've asked for help and stayed sober for a few days. So why are my emotions still so intense?

Change can feel uncomfortable. Do you mind if we discuss feeling banished a bit more?

It's kind of embarrassing, but I guess so.

I understand. I'll be kind. What's the Unreliable Narrator saying right now?

My Unreliable Narrator says I don't belong.

And?

And that I never will.

And you want to numb out?

I do want to numb out.

To the Survival Brain, numbing out seems like a shelter from the old familiar tapes of the Unreliable Narrator.

Now I'm berating myself for believing the Unreliable Narrator. Drinking does feel like taking shelter, like a reprieve, a break, a refuge.

Maybe for a few moments. It's easy to forget consequences when seeking shelter seems urgent. Berating yourself obscures your ability to look at yourself more honestly. You can ease up.

Is there a support group for self-flagellation?

Good idea. For now, I'll have you Write the Scene.

Another skill?

Another skill.

Write the scene you're living right now as if you're a playwright. Give the scene detail. Help the audience feel the character's emotions. Where is she? If she's in the 3F Red Zone or the Yellow Caution Zone, show how that feels. If not, skip that part. Take a few Spare Tire Breaths. What is spinning in her mind? Give the scene a title. Is her mind looping? Does it feel uplifting or restrictive or repetitive? Describe the physical sensations, the tension, and each emotion. Get tactile. Include the set, the floor, the fabrics, the drape of her clothing, the smell of the linens. Pop me in the scene for a bit of helpful feedback.

Okay, here goes. I'll call this scene…

The Swamp of Temptation and Banishment

A woman makes fists and play-acts punching herself unconscious. In dim grey tones, she sits in a hotel bed next to her sleeping boyfriend. The opposite side of the stage, divided by a wall, shows a pool and a bar with lively people having a grand time with colorful string lights, palm trees, and balloons.

                THE UNRELIABLE NARRATOR.
                    (off stage.)
            "Go have fun. Who will know?"

                        SIL.
                (whispers defiantly.)
            "Be quiet. I'm on to you."

Sil sits up and loudly takes a few Spare Tire Breaths. She massages her neck, shoulders, and jaw muscles and winces in pain as if the tightness is cemented in place, dense, weighty, and intractable. She stands up and pulls invisible swords from her side and with an angry face, she swings and thrusts the swords in an imaginary fight. She falls in defeat and lifts her arms against the blows from her unseen opponent. She brings her hands to her face and screams a silent scream.

Offstage a scuffle is heard, and a new voice speaks.

> CAVE WOMAN.
> (off stage.)
> "You're doing great. Release the rage and fear a little at a time. No need to blow everything up again. Remember, swamps can be healthy, too. Go in the bathroom and take a few Volcano Breaths. Listen to some recovery stories online. I'll sit with you all night."

Sil does as Cave Woman suggests, returns to bed, puts on her headphones, leans back, and sighs.

Bravo!

That's it?

How do you feel now?

Better. Oh, I see. I stepped back from the moment and saw things from a slightly different perspective. Like I was mediating between the various aspects of myself. Very clever.

Mediating is a good word. I knew you'd like "Write the Scene."

I think adding some melodrama helped me smile a little.

I do too. Now what?

Now, I listen to a recovery story online.

Mumbo Jumbo

Dear Cave Woman,

I'm back. It's the middle of the night and I still can't sleep. I listened to recovery stories online, but I can't concentrate anymore. I feel raw like I'm standing naked in a howling sandstorm. I'm hating myself and worried.

Let worry know you're doing what it takes to stay in recovery.

Emotions are hard to ignore without drinking.

You can put off feeling emotions for a time, but you can't ignore them entirely. Give your worry some attention and unruffle its feathers before it takes full flight into panic.

But I felt good earlier. The meetings helped. You helped. Cole helped. Now I feel guilty because I'm worrying again. I don't really believe in religious scaremongering, and this is embarrassing, but am I being punished for my past mistakes?

You're not being punished. If you could hear your fear over the blare of self-hatred, it would tell you that what happened propelled you into recovery.

Can we just stick with the practical stuff and lay off the spiritual mumbo jumbo?

We can as long as the practical stuff is useful. The world is paradoxical. The more interesting aspects of life often defy logic, which makes each day compelling.

Chapter 10

Shake me Down

Even though I didn't sleep, I got up and attended an early morning meeting. Afterward, I asked a kindly woman older than myself if she'd take me on as a sponsee. She turned me down. My voice shook so much I nearly shouted to get the words out. She said she and her wife both have health challenges, and she couldn't take on anything else right now. I said I understood, but it hurt my feelings. I felt the familiar din of rejection.

As I drove back to the hotel, my mind replayed times I felt rejected; my first boyfriend having an affair, a best friend moving away, the older kids in the neighborhood excluding me, a C on a college paper I thought was pretty damn good, people dismissing concerns about my mom. I breathed into my spare tire and I felt better, but I still feel nervous asking anyone else about sponsoring me.

When I get back, Cole isn't in our room. I eat the last piece of a leftover pizza and wish I had an entire pizza. I consider buying snacks at the gift shop, but the idea of walking past the party by the pool makes me tired.

I don't want to cry, but I do and it's painful, like I've swallowed a rusty tin can filled with old bolts and nails. I try stopping but can't. I lurch around the room looking for a distraction. I lay on the floor and let the tears shake me down.

I find my Cave Woman notebook and crawl in bed, fully clothed.

—⚋—

Dear Cave Woman,

How did you recover when your feelings were hurt? How did others in your community deal with rejection?

We'd fall down or fall apart. We'd cry or throw a tantrum, just like you did today. Laughter also helped us express feelings. Emotional displays were commonplace in my community and never shocked us; it was expected.

Besides, a good cloudburst can help clear hidden debris.

I feel like an old science fiction octopus. One tentacle reaches for a bottle propelled by an evil storyteller, one tentacle reaches for a bottle to avoid feelings, one tentacle reaches for a bottle to ignore survival responses. How can I remember all this, much less handle the next craving?

You're already handling each craving. You're remembering. It's been a long time since you went a few weeks without alcohol. You're moving emotional energy and clearing the stuck sediment. You're noticing the Unreliable Narrator and changing outdated patterns.

Okay, let's see if we can change a bit more of the narration now. I need encouragement.

What else am I doing right?

You're beginning to discern an emotional flashback from a current emotion. You're recognizing how the Yellow Caution

Zone feels. You're hurting when you're hurt and enjoying a few moments here and there and you're talking to me.

You're not arguing with the discomfort.

Why is that important?

You're learning more about the human experience and not taking the ups and downs so personally. Most importantly, you're resting and playing.

Why does that matter?

During rest and play, the work you've done takes hold. Bread only rises when the kneading stops.

I feel like I'm all over the map.

I know my fidgety hummingbird.

This is easy for you. All you do is talk in my head. I don't think you know what it's like to live in my world. Sounds like your people had a great rapport. We don't have that.

No, you don't, not to the extent my people did, but you could have a close approximation by developing a rapport with yourself. You've already started by not always fighting what's happening internally. You won't be as shocked as things come up and neither will your nervous system. People won't baffle you quite as much. You won't baffle yourself quite as much. Remember to remain curious and accept kindness if offered.

I don't even know how to accept a gift graciously, much less ask for help. I did that today and got turned down.

You asked me for help. I'm sorry that you learned asking for help is wrong, but it can be unlearned. Just by communicating with me, you're practicing receiving, which will help you notice messages from your emotions, your intuition, and from the whole damn universe.

Asking for help terrifies me. My heart pounds just thinking

about asking someone else to be my sponsor. I know fear has value but surely not to this extreme.

If someone asked you for help and you didn't have the time, would you want that person to judge themselves as worthless?

No.

Give it time and keep taking turtle steps. Remember, everyone who has overcome an addiction feared asking for help. Modern culture blames addiction on the individual, but addiction is a societal problem. Overcoming a drinking habit will help heal other habits as well. The human species needs to know healing is possible.

Recovery is not just about you.

Can I just stay in bed forever? Can you hand me the TV remote?

You've always wanted to stage a revolution, helping humans and animals regain both respect and justice. Break the trance of old societal conditioning. Risk the embarrassment and keep asking for help. It's rebellious.

I want to ride with rebels and dethrone tyrants, not sit in my own shame. This is not my idea of revolution. I need a break.

All This Damn Shame

I hit the vending machine. Two hours and three bags of potato chips later, Cole still isn't back. I don't want to call and make him think I don't trust him. It's humankind I don't trust. Cole is like the doe-eyed nice guy in the movie who gets killed first. I wish he was back. I wish I could let him have some time alone without needing him so much. I wish I trusted myself.

—ɯ—

Dear Cave Woman,

I depend on Cole too much. He's my rock and I cling to him like moss. I'm so ashamed, I don't want to talk about it. What else can we talk about?

Tell me more about your mom.

Okay, this is the first thing that comes to mind:

My mom and I read hundreds of books together even though we lived a thousand miles apart. We'd wait until each of us had a copy from the library to start reading. My mom usually read a book in less than a week, but she'd take notes while I caught up. One time, we read a book about a mother and child who were separated at the Mexican border. It's not clear at the end if they were reunited. On the phone, my mom's voice, thick with tears, asked me if I thought they'd reunite. I assured her they would. I think I lied.

You thought the mother and child would reunite, which was simply your opinion. You didn't lie. Tell me about visiting your mom during the heat wave.

I visited my Mom in DC the summer after her fall. My dad left to go to their cabin in Montana, and I agreed to stay with her for two weeks. When I arrived, the air conditioning was broken, and the humidity and temperature hovered in the upper nineties.

She seemed suspicious of me. She could play the part and say the right things, but she was more like an actor playing my mom than my mom. Her own mother had devolved into dementia with extreme paranoia. She ended up catatonic, sitting straight up in bed at a mental institution for the last years of her life. I hadn't realized the extent of my mom's brain damage until I saw her in person. My mom could act as if everything was fine much better on the phone than in person.

A few days before I left, she accused me of conspiring against her when I told her Dad would be coming back. I wasn't shocked anymore, just heartbroken and missing the woman who sat in the bed next to me. The shock would come a few years later when the worst heartbreak of my life escalated into a nightmare I never saw coming. I thought—

—⚮—

Cole opens the hotel door and I jump up and hug him and smash the big bag of warm burritos he's carrying. "I hope you don't mind," he says, pointing to the bag. "I ate some tacos at a little Mexican place. The tacos were so good, I picked up dinner to go."

"I don't mind," I say, grinning and taking the bag from him.

We turn on some lights and sit down on the faded green couch to eat. I would have liked to take a shower before dinner. The shame I felt for being turned down by a potential sponsor, the shame at needing Cole, and the shame of being an inept helper for my mom all have me feeling rumpled and sweaty. Instead, I add extra hot sauce and act like the spice is making me sweat.

Cole tells me about his day-long walk. He says he's having fun and I need to stop worrying so much. I tell him I'd hoped he wouldn't notice, but I'm getting there.

We watch TV and Cole falls asleep on the couch. I get in bed just a few feet away and decide to ask Cave Woman about all this damn shame.

—⚮—

Dear Cave Woman,

Where does all this shame come from? Why is shame so unrelenting? I know you said asking for help is rebellious, and I like that, but I still break out in a shame sweat just thinking about being so needy.

You're experiencing a great deal of shame from difficulties in your childhood and echoes of shame from your parents, grandparents, and even further back.

Without healthy and wise communities, trauma travels like a stowaway through family lines. Addiction thrives in places where asking for help is deemed shameful.

Addiction masks shame momentarily but can never resolve shame. Shame needs you to hear its message.

I've felt shame every day of my entire life. When I was young, I was very bold and friendly, but later I felt embarrassed to be alive. I tried to hide in big black coats. My brain felt hot when I had to speak. I'd get dizzy and even fainted a few times. Now shame rules me.

If shame causes such problems, why does it exist?

Healthy shame reminds us to reconnect with our inner hive, other human beings, and to a world outside our own thoughts. Shame reminded me when I'd done something or experienced something that could separate me from my community. Shame reminded me to keep reaching out until I found a heartfelt connection.

You told people when you felt shame? How embarrassing.

To tell someone I felt shame was to tell them I felt disconnected. Shame warned me that my connection had waned and my job, often with help, was to plug back in.

A little shame sounds helpful. I get it. But the shame I feel is stupefying like I'm wearing a bodysuit filled with hot peppers.

Except for your father, expressing anger was unacceptable in your family. Being denied anger left you without a healthy perimeter.

Why was shame acceptable but not anger?

There are two reasons. Firstly, shame was not only acceptable, it was cultivated as a means of control to keep you compliant.

And secondly?

Secondly, shame became a decoy to distract you from expressing anger which could've led to more violence and abuse. This is called Decoy Shame.

But I feel a lot of anger inside. Rage even. But I do feel shame whenever I feel angry and that makes me so mad. I can feel the shame ebbing away just by getting mad. Can I get rid of shame altogether?

No, you still need shame. What you don't need is Decoy Shame preventing you from feeling and using your healthy anger to set safe perimeters.

Decoy shame is like channel where other emotions get diverted?

That's a good analogy. Other emotions use the shame channel because its wide open. When you feel shame ask if you're mad, sad, glad, or afraid. See what other emotion is using the shame channel. Feeling that other emotion separately will lessen the Decoy Shame.

No wonder I have so much shame. Shame is doing double duty. My perimeters are made of apologies for being alive, which lets anyone trample all over me.

Yes, shame was trained as a decoy to turn you away from anger.

How can I possibly express all the anger that was left unvoiced?

Write down the rage a little at a time.

That will take forever.

And I'll be here forever.

Can you say more about the useful side of shame? I don't feel so blindsided when you tell me the benefits of emotions.

I'm glad. I want you to see emotions as ordinary and having a useful purpose.

Emotions are specific to each person, but here are a few general thoughts about why shame—not decoy shame—can be useful:

Shame propels you to get help. You wouldn't be in recovery without shame.

Shame lets you see where you've lost your own sense of decency and redirects you to regain your bearings. You wouldn't be writing to me without shame.

Shame informs you when you have something to make up for or owe an apology to yourself or others. You wouldn't be reuniting your inner hive without shame.

Shame reminds you to enlist your self-regard. Ask yourself, "How am I doing with this situation? Am I okay, or am I freaking out? Am I calm, jumpy, tense? All three?" Self-regard pulls you out of the internal chaos spun by the Unreliable Narrator and reminds you to check for actual hazards.

I've heard self-love is part of healing. If you're tricking me into loving myself, don't waste your time.

I might be. Who knows? My people were like gyroscopes. We were constantly adjusting our inner world to stay aligned with well-being. Self-regard was, and still is, invaluable.

If I understand correctly, shame is helping me to stay in recovery and do what I can to repair the damage I've caused.

That's right, my little larvae. Your inner community is composed of every note in the universe and every song ever written. To lead your inner community, you have intellect, all your senses, including common sense, all kinds of languages, including body language, musical language, the music of language—written or spoken or signed—including cadence and rhythm, the language of the body, and the ability to move through space and time.

I'm not musical.

Language is musical. If you could turn your cynicism down just one degree, the world would shift its axis.

I still wish I never had to feel shame again. It's very uncomfortable.

Be damn glad you do. The people among you who feel no shame are the most dangerous animals on Earth. They believe they have the right to harm whomever they choose. Those without shame exploit and manipulate others. Appreciate the value of healthy shame.

Let me tell you a story.

A young couple looking for a hiding place to kiss each other got stuck high up in a tree. Their excitement to be together propelled them like monkeys up a trunk they couldn't scale back down. The height seemed much further after an hour of kissing than it did when they'd clambered up the branches.

We didn't look for them until nightfall. We fanned out in a circle and then came back together. We'd move a few hundred feet and fan out again. I imagined the patterns we were making as if seen by a bird.

The traces of our movements made lovely art. I was fascinated by all the traces left by the natural world. Shifting rivers, animal migrations, snail trails, eddies in water, scorch marks on firewood, salt crystals, how the wind and sand play and settle into temporary masterpieces. And even how people die and come back to life, which happened in my community. I didn't see it myself, but I'd heard about it plenty of times. They always came back with insights that made our lives better.

The young man decided to shimmy down the tree, but he lost his grip and fell to his death. Seeing her beloved lying dead on the ground, the young woman jumped without a moment's thought to join him in the next life. She chose to die rather than face life without him. The blush of new love often causes impulsivity. And foolishness. She miscalculated the jump and landed directly on her beloved, breaking her fall. In death, his body saved her life. Instead of relief, she felt horrified by his lifeless body. She felt great shame that the man she couldn't get enough of a few moments ago now repelled her. And ashamed she couldn't show proper respect and failed to join him in death. She believed she would be banished if she returned to our hive and ran away from our community.

She ran without looking where she was going, hoping death would take her unaware so she couldn't avoid it again. She had heard of people who can escape death over and over. She wanted to live and die at the same time. She cried and stumbled, got up and cried and stumbled again and again.

She stopped for a moment and considered returning to us, but she was too ashamed. She couldn't face admitting her failure to die with her beloved. She howled and knew she couldn't admit her repulsion at his lifeless body. She resolved to banish herself until Mother Earth opened and swallowed her whole.

Her panic kept her running away from her hive and further into certain death. She had never been alone before but worry kept her from seeking our counsel. Her panic only grew.

Next to the tree, the young man coughed and sputtered back to life. Maybe his heart had stopped on impact, and the young woman's fall had restarted his heart. Perhaps he'd just been knocked unconscious. Regardless, he woke early in the morning to find her gone. He panicked, found her tracks, and started to follow. He assumed his ineptness at getting out of the tree and knocking himself out made her run off in disgust. Realizing her tracks were going away from our hive, he worried she may not have survived the night. The shame of his own incompetence pained his bruised heart. He resolved to find her even if she was no longer alive.

On the second morning, a group of us set out again to find them. We found the tree and saw in the dirt what looked like traces of a scuffle. But there were no drag marks and no blood. It looked like one person had run off, and the other had followed.

Our shame-crossed lovers continued to run away from the comfort and safety of our community.

We could feel they were still alive, but we also felt their panic. We settled ourselves to track them. One community member, in a vision, saw a large rock near a familiar spring. He saw both the young man and the young woman meeting there, surprised to see each other. This confused us since we'd assumed they'd been together the whole time.

When we arrived, we found the young woman asleep beside the rock. She wept and seemed reluctant to tell us what happened. She could barely speak. The group told her they would sit and rest and then look for the young man.

The young man approached the group, shocked to see his beloved. The young woman was equally shocked. Having assumed the other was dead, they approached each other like ghosts, unsure the other was real. When they finally understood they were both still flesh and blood, they embraced and thanked our community for finding them before their foolishness caused even more chaos and despair.

As we returned home, the young couple's story came to light. We knew their tale could've ended tragically, but many of us had difficulty hiding our laughter. The poor couple looked horrified at our giggling. We apologized and attempted to remain serious. But, over the years, the story got funnier with each retelling until the lovers themselves could laugh, too. They ended up repeating their story countless times, so much so that it became a parable. Their story came to illustrate that if you sit with shame long enough, and don't run away, what you love most in the world will return.

Chapter 11

True Kinship

I'm at the library sitting in a boxy yellow leather chair. It might be Naugahyde; I'm not sure, but it stays soft and quiet when I fidget.

Maybe I'm not allowed to sit here without a library card, but so far, everyone ignores me. I stopped here to write to Cave Woman after a meeting and gather my thoughts. I won't stay long.

At the meeting, a group of women arrived in a van from a rehab center. Several of them spoke and said they chose rehab over jail. One woman's nephew and aunt died in a car accident. All the adults in the car were drunk. She didn't say who was driving, but it was instantly clear to everyone in the room that it didn't matter. It could have been any one of us. A chill ran through the room.

Dear Cave Woman,

I'm still having trouble talking with people before or after the meetings. I have this strange idea I need to confess and talk about what I'm most ashamed of, which violates the rules I grew up with. I want to talk with people in recovery more. I want to reach out more. Instead, the moment the meeting ends, I usually dash to my car. Everyone else talks to each other, but I run. I can't stay. I don't know if I can trust these people with my darkest secrets.

Give yourself credit for going to meetings at all. You're changing even if you don't realize it yet. Please don't berate yourself for not undergoing a difficult change more perfectly.

I feel afraid but it's not stopping me from going.

Yes, see? That's different than the fear you'd feel if it wasn't safe to be there at all.

Are you afraid of these people?

I'm afraid, period. I don't think I'm afraid of them specifically. With every story I hear, I wonder why we continue to drink despite such terrible consequences.

Alcohol causes people to override good sense. People also feel kinship when they consume alcohol. Even drinking alone feels like community. It's a seductive illusion. While alcohol does create similar feelings I had with my hive, those feelings are fleeting.

Alcohol does get people to do things that they wouldn't otherwise.

Which leaves many people feeling shame because the sober light of day exposes the betrayal. Then people return to bars and parties because they still long for genuine connection. The longing signifies a capacity for true kinship.

You mean being an alcoholic is a sign that I long for genuine connection? If that's true, why do I feel shame talking about this addiction?

You were taught—tragically—that needing other people is embarrassing. Yet, humans are born needing care and

remain in need of care. **Caring for each other is how my community survived.**

If I had the time and a better memory, I bet I could list a million times when I stopped myself from asking for help because I feared rejection.

You felt banished from your family, like you were broken and worthy of rejection. You thought that you were an unwanted person, unworthy and undeserving. Continuing to feel defective is far riskier than saying hello to someone after a meeting. The risk of continuing to feel that way is far greater than reaching out to a sober community.

Should I talk more about old traumas and what I do remember to clear out the old stuff?

Hashed out on paper and with another living human who makes you feel heard is a good start. Find a trustworthy human, look them in the eye, and tell the truth about what happened in your life. When we feel heard, our life story fades as a cause for cravings. We gain perspective and create a new script.

I keep hearing at meetings that insanity is doing the same thing over and over again, expecting a different result. I think they're talking about addiction.

And it didn't ring true for you?

No, I drank precisely to have a predictable experience of my feelings.

I agree. You could predict how you felt for a time and remove the Unreliable Narrator's sting. With understanding and practice, you'll feel less awkward around new people.

I keep hearing at meetings that I need to surrender. Why do I need to surrender?

You surrender the old narration and admit it never worked for you. You surrender to the task of writing a new script with

your Creative Genius. When you surrender, you surrender the obvious fact that alcohol is not your hive, never has been and never will be.

You mentioned we'd talk more about intuition.

Ah, your memory is improving! Your intuition, your inner knowing, urges you to connect with a sober community to help re-forge the bond that was lost many generations ago.

Your stumbling, bumbling, and vulnerability helps others.

Maybe I could keep my mouth shut until I feel better?

Didn't someone tell you to just listen for now and not speak at meetings?

Oh yeah, I forgot. Several people said newbies should just listen for the first month. Here I am putting all this pressure on myself to talk when I've been told to listen.

You put a great deal of pressure on yourself. You have for a very long time. It's a habit that we'll ease together.

Your instinct to connect is healthy. Please know that disconnection happens and reconnection—healthy reconnection—is possible.

Fasten your seat belt, my precious kakapo, it's not a pretty landing, but you will survive.

It sounds like you think I'll stay sober.

Why would I assume anything other than what your heart truly desires?

Odell

I meet Cole for lunch and then he drops me off at a women's meeting. After the meeting, two women approach me as I attempt to sneak out.

"We're having a potluck at my house tonight. It's part meeting, part potluck, and you're coming. I'm Odell, this is Jane," says a formidable woman with sun-weathered skin the color of a saddle. Jane stands next to her in a long flowery dress, smiling and shaking her head yes.

"Thank you but I can't. I get sick in the evenings; nauseous and dizzy and I have to lie down."

"Too bad," Odell says. "You're coming. Take a cab if you have to. Skip bringing a dish. There'll be plenty of food."

I open my mouth to protest, but she interrupts and says, "Do you have someone to help navigate sobriety yet?"

"No," I say suspiciously.

"You do now. Give me that notebook sticking out of your back-pack." She writes her number on the back of my notebook and hands it back.

I examine what Odell wrote and when I look up, they're already walking away.

"See you tonight!" shouts Odell.

Jane smiles and gives me a thumbs up.

Cole arrives to pick me up and asks what's wrong.

"Nothing, why?" I ask, distracted.

Cole looks at me and says, "You look like you're in shock."

"I met someone who's going to help me one-on-one with sobriety. Have you ever felt ambushed by an offer of help?" I ask.

"Not really but it sounds kind of nice, actually."

"You know, you're right. It was nice. I needed a push. Her name is Odell and I'm going to her house tonight for a potluck dinner with a bunch of other women."

"I love potluck dinners. I remember all the Italian women cooking suppers in the church basement. The food was so good. This is making me hungry. You're lucky."

"You know what, I think you're right."

Have a Seat

I've decided to drive myself to Odell's instead of having Cole drop me off or taking a cab. I want to make a quick exit if I feel overwhelmed.

I'm nervous and nauseous. I park and get out of the car quickly before I change my mind. The door is ajar, so I step inside but freeze. Should I have knocked? Odell yells from the kitchen, "Make yourself at home, have a seat."

The house smells like a vet's office. There are animals everywhere. Cats on bookcases, dogs wrestling inside a circle of mismatched chairs in the living room, goats bleating outside, and an animal who darts down a hallway so fast, I can't identify it.

About ten women converse like they all know each other well. No room for me. I turn around and reach for the door handle.

"Not so fast. Get over here and sit by me," I hear Odell say as she walks toward me. "You'll be okay. We've all felt as crappy as you do right now."

"I, I, I...doubt that," I stammer. Everyone laughs and returns to their conversations. I feel humiliated. My legs feel rubbery and the heat from my chest hikes up my neck. I sit where there's a clear path to the front door if I need to run outside and hurl. I pet several ecstatic and drooling dogs who act like they've never been petted before, taking turns making me feel needed. If there's food, I can't smell it over the vet-office aroma.

"Quiet down now. We've got a newbie and we don't need to act like a bunch of cackling chickens. Let's get this done so this poor woman can escape our clutches."

They laugh at me. I look at the floor and the room falls quiet.

The women take turns sharing their lives over the past month.

One woman with bright clear eyes, a nurse, celebrated twenty years in sobriety. She's excited about a big promotion at the hospital. She's friendly and full of laughter. I couldn't imagine her ever being anything other than fully pulled together and accomplished. We hear from a mechanic, a chef, a grandma, a judge, and a woman dressed all in purple, her forearms loaded with jangly bracelets. There are tears, setbacks, and new perspectives gained.

My turn comes and I say, "This past month I moved, and I drank. But then I meet people like the women here tonight. Next month I'm kind of hoping to keep moving and skip the drinking part."

They laugh at me again.

I add, "That's all," and get up and find the bathroom. Luckily, the first door I open in the narrow hallway is the bathroom. What a relief. I sit on the toilet and notice two litter boxes in the bathtub. The smell doesn't help my nausea. I'm either going to cry or throw up. I settle on crying but only a few tears fall. I'd sneak out, but there's no window. I hear the chairs squeaking on the wood floor and the roar of conversation begins again. I guess it's time to eat.

I blow my nose and wash my face with a tiny trickle of water from a stingy faucet and return to the living room. Odell brings me a plate of food and some water. The food's good. I've never had three different casseroles at one time. The comfort food eases my nausea. I drink the lukewarm water and tell Odell I really need to leave.

She says, "Okay. You got here and that's what counts. You're not going to do something stupid on the way home, are you?"

"No," I say and mean it. I have no desire to drink and I'm not sure why.

"Call me in the morning," Odell insists.

"I will, thank you for everything," I say and make my exit, relieved to have made my first foray into the world without the promise of wine as a reward.

Back at the hotel, Cole asks, "How was your party?"

"Good," I say, "really interesting actually." My answer surprises me. I thought I'd regret going but I don't. Instead, I feel kind of peppy.

Unique to You

I'm buzzing from being around so many people. Is this how optimism feels? My chest and stomach feel like I drank a fizzy soda too fast. Optimism seems dangerous and my mind whirrs and creates a list of my past misdeeds and past disappointments. I'm not sure even Cave Woman can help, but I'll ask her anyway since I'm awake and Cole's asleep.

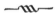

Dear Cave Woman,

I think about the past a lot and obsess about what I could have done differently. That kind of fear isn't at all useful. It's awful.

What if fear is urging you to let the past remain in the past?

Ask fear what I need to focus on now?

Exactly. What answer did you get?

The emotion is not the message. The emotion contains a message.

Beautiful. What else?

The messages are not always what we would assume. Is that accurate?

That's correct.

For example?

For example, sadness might tell you it's okay to leave and move on or tell you to hold on because things are looking up.

Confusion might tell you to take a break from the problem you're working so hard to solve.

Panic might ask you to hear your own advice.

Anxiety might encourage you to get ready for what's next.

Fear might remind you to not give a damn what anyone thinks and follow your own guidance.

Jealousy might invite you to love yourself more.

Emotions bring specific messages that you may not expect. Think about my take on emotions as training wheels. Eventually, you'll view them through the lens of your own intuition.

I think I understand. I'll get my own unique messages the more I practice feeling emotions.

Yes, and I can promise you this; If the message is not helpful, you're hearing your mind chatter and not the emotion.

The Unreliable Narrator reading from the old script again?

Mind chatter can jump in and give you a scary or disturbing message, which you'll find decidedly unhelpful.

If the message helps you and brings relief or insight, it's the emotion talking.

Can't you just blink your eyes or wave your hands and make me better? Where's my fairy godmother when I need her?

Maybe emotions are your fairy godmother. Ask them. I can't make you see your own wholeness in an instant. If I could, I would. But I promise you're becoming more...

Wholeier?

Nice play on words.

But I don't believe––

It doesn't matter whether you believe your 'wholeiness' consists of the cells in your body, a rapture of angels, Venus and Jupiter, a feeling of awe, a better left brain/right brain

**balance, orange trees, elephant seals, or the insights each life
leaves for you to pluck from the Creative Genius.**
    Do you think you can rest for a while?
    Maybe I'll listen to something online. I might be back.
    I'm here.

—⟋⟍—

Dust and Dog Hair

Odell is an urban farmer with goats, chickens, ducks, cats, dogs, and a large sunken kiddie pool filled with tilapia. I've spent the last three mornings at her house, talking. Today we sit on her front porch behind a veil of climbing clematis grown to help keep the house cooler. It's not very hot yet, but it makes a nice fort. We can see out but remain largely hidden from those passing by. I like hiding from the slings and arrows of critical eyes. It's hiding from my own built-in brutal critic that's the trick. But it's nothing I don't deserve.

Odell talks, skillfully ignoring the squawking ducks and bleating goats. "It's your job to contact me. I'm not your babysitter. Understood?" she asks.

"Understood," I confirm but my attention wanders from what she's saying. I'm fighting with myself. I'm not sure if I should tell her what I did. I'm afraid if I tell her, I'll drink. I'm afraid if I keep quiet any longer, I'll drink. I'm afraid she'll hate me when she finds out. Here on this little farm, in a neighborhood of small, single-family homes, I feel like a traitor to the animal kingdom. I don't let her speak for long before I interrupt and confess about leaving Maddy.

"I abandoned my cat," I blurt out. Tears twist my throat, but I keep talking. "She was like my daughter. I left her to get away. To take a job that may not even happen. It's the worst thing I've ever done. I didn't know I could do anything this horrible."

Odell tosses me a box of tissues covered with dust and dog hair.

"I swore all my life I wouldn't pass down what was done to me. No one would be abandoned. I thought I'd skipped that by not having children. But, oh crap, I did it anyway. I can't live knowing I abandoned my baby."

I want Odell to kick me off her property or feed me to her animals as retribution.

But she just nods her head and says, "Addiction takes everything. It even takes who you thought you were. Regret and resentment are killers. Are you ready to stay sober?"

Odell doesn't mince words.

"Yes," I promise, and I mean it. "For Maddy."

I feel tapped out and we fall silent for a time.

Odell breaks the silence and asks, "Would you and Cole have time to help me move some rocks around the duck pond? It's an old cattle tank and I'd like to pile up some large rocks so the ducks can perch closer to the water."

"That's such a normal request, not something you would ask the worst person on Earth."

"No, it's not. Can you call Cole now?"

I gently tug my backpack out from under a large black dog, find my phone, and call Cole.

I go to the hotel and pick him up and we work in the sun for a few hours. Cole enjoys doing something productive and asks Odell about each animal and her energy-efficiency experiments. I can tell she loves sharing all the details, but the heat starts to make me dizzy.

"I need to get out of the sun and lay down for a while," I say, but they keep talking. Leaving always takes time so I let them continue for about fifteen minutes before insisting.

"Okay, can we go now?" I sound whiney and I don't care.

Odell laughs and helps me out by saying, "Get outta here you two."

We head back to our hotel past the University of Arizona, and several bars and liquor stores. The "Cold Beer" signs look bright and inviting and my mouth waters. The air conditioning is slow to cool the sunbaked car and sweat trickles down our faces. I reach for my water bottle and find it empty. My mouth feels dry, but a deeper thirst wants attention.

In the past, I'd made Cole pick up alcohol for me on his way home from work when I'd already started drinking and didn't want to drive. Cole always accommodated. He has a hard time saying no to anyone.

"Are you ready to get some beer?" The words slip out of my mouth before I can think, slick as a wet pile of pebbles.

"No," Cole says. His adamant reply surprises us both.

"Ice cream?" I ask, attempting to save face. We just spent an afternoon with the person helping me stay sober and I'd nearly made him complicit in my drinking again.

"Yes," he states evenly.

We stop for soft-serve cones with sprinkles.

As we leave the drive-thru, I say, "Thank you."

We both know it's not about the ice cream.

Chapter 12

Speaker Meeting

In a lonely but bright corner of a cavernous church basement, six rows of folding chairs sit in six neat rows. I worry the florescent lights showcase the dark circles under my eyes. At seven days sober, I feel like a dilapidated house that's too far gone to bother fixing up. Regrets tramp through my stomach. I still haven't slept and don't know how long a person can live without sleep. I'm falling apart from the inside out.

As I cross the room, I feel a panic attack begin. It feels as if my soul is leaking out of my body onto the yellow speckled linoleum floor. I squeeze my shoulders, attempting to keep mind and soul paired until I reach my seat.

I sit in an aisle seat in the back row and gingerly set my iced tea by the side of the metal folding chair so when I fall over dead it won't spill and make a mess.

The woman sitting beside me seems to know I'm new and leans over and whispers loudly, "This is what's called a speaker meeting. At speaker meetings someone is asked in advance to share their story for twenty or thirty minutes and then we're free to talk after that."

I hope the speaker doesn't take me dropping dead personally. "Oh, good, that leaves me less time to remain awkwardly silent," I joke.

The woman frowns and leans back in her chair. I guess I could attempt to dampen my cynicism a little.

The speaker stands with her arms crossed in an ironed white shirt, creased green cargo pants, and a wide leather belt. She begins to pace as the chairwoman introduces her. We are an audience of about twenty-five souls. Her ramrod-straight back makes me wonder if she's military.

She starts, "My father brought the war home to my family. After his return, my two older brothers, who had been my protectors, became my tormentors. Dad chased them around the outside of the house yelling things that made no sense. He shouted at them to run because they could be killed at any minute by no-good whores, or by the enemy, or by my father himself, if they didn't listen and toughen up quick."

I reach for my iced tea and take a long drink. I'm interested in her story and my soul and body reunite to listen more closely. I'd grown up quasi-military; meaning my Dad's government job gave us some military benefits like access to the PX, commissary, and hospitals. The military hospital part rarely felt like a benefit. Seeing a doctor usually meant spending the better part of a day waiting in a hard-plastic chair, in the hallway of a nineteenth-century brick building that resembled a horror movie asylum.

I didn't mind the waiting part. With time on our hands, my mom told me stories from her childhood. She always had stories to tell. Her parents went looking for work during the Great Depression and left her alone at fifteen years old. She made it sound like an adventure instead of tragedy.

I also watched my mom talk with seemingly forgotten Vietnam vets parked on gurneys in the long, moss-green hallways. She spoke with them about the latest book she'd discovered or an interesting item she'd read in the paper. Like Fibonacci numbers and the golden triangle and how everything in nature, including flowers, grows and forms in specific patterns. How the eye finds these patterns pleasing and that's what we call beauty. Or she might talk about an Aboriginal art exhibit and how the Aboriginals spoke of things that had happened 50,000 years ago—passed accurately through an inconceivable number of generations. Stories archeologists confirm as historically accurate.

Most of the people waiting for appointments ignored the veterans. My mom found topics each vet would find interesting. Or maybe she just knew what not to talk about, like war and politics. I was sick a lot, which meant we spent many hours waiting in eerie hospital hallways, as I watched injured young men light up and fall for my kindhearted mom.

I take a sip from my iced tea again and enjoy the coolness on my throat. I look at the floor and focus on her words, which relieves the dizziness.

"I learned to hide, I had to. I learned to run. I learned to stay alert even when I slept, which was rare. School became a nightmare. I was too tired to pay attention. When I fell asleep in class, I begged them not to call home. I knew what would happen when I got back to the house.

"Our mother could take our father's attention away from us for a time with alcohol and pot. She had my brothers buy drugs and give them to my father to help knock him out. It rarely worked. His adrenaline levels had been left on full blast. They all started drinking every day. Food was scarce. I taught myself to fish, but the cooking fire gave away my position, which put an end to that. I started foraging for quieter dinners.

"I don't blame my brothers for abusing me. I don't even blame my dad. I blame the war and everyone and everything that led up to it. I blame every war. I blame people for believing hateful lies about other people enough to kill them. I blame myself, which I'm told I was taught to do. My therapist said healing takes time.

"I work long hours by choice. I need to stay busy. I've been diagnosed with PTSD and working a lot is the only way I can burn all the restless energy inside of me. It's the only way I can get any sleep at all. For now, working is one way I can manage my symptoms.

"With the help of all of you and my sponsor, I'm sober now, too. Drinking gave me some relief from my symptoms but made the nightmarish parts of my life much worse. Recovery has saved my life. I'm thankful for that. At the same time, I look forward to how much more recovery has in store for me and many more like me." She stopped pacing, faced the group, and said, "Now, the hard part."

That wasn't the hard part?

"This is the first time I've told my story. Yes, I was nervous. Yes, I had a difficult time walking into this building today. I've never wanted to tell my story before. I know some of you will line up to speak with me, which is fine, but some of you will want hugs. I can't take being touched. I apologize. I'm just not there yet and I may never be. Thank you for respecting that."

We clap, which I'd never heard at a recovery meeting before. It felt right.

I want to hug her tight and push away her nightmarish past. Barring that, I resolve to thank her because I now know, without a doubt, that I have PTSD, too. I'm constantly on high alert and needed alcohol for sleep. My mind could run the same thought a million times until I drank to shut it up. I treated panic attacks with wine. I'd taken antidepressants, which never had a chance since alcohol acts as a depressant.

After hearing her story, my rising panic attack diminished completely. I'm nervous but I risk talking to her directly. After the meeting, I approach her and blurt out, "I didn't have it nearly as bad as you did." We look each other in the eye, and we both immediately look away. But I feel safe with her and I know it doesn't matter how awkwardly I speak. Small talk isn't necessary. "But I think I have some PTSD, too," I add.

She hugs herself and replies, "It's not a matter of degrees it's a matter of if. If there was childhood trauma, there will be PTSD. When you understand, you can begin to heal. Trying to minimize it will only make your life hell on Earth."

I thank her and walk away. For the first time, I don't feel embarrassed leaving a conversation without exchanging phone numbers or making a promise to get together. We understood each other and that's enough.

Ghost Writer

Cole's working with Michael, the man we met at Denny's, building a gadget for a movie set. I asked for details, but he said it was complicated. I haven't seen him this excited about a project in a long time. We used to build tiny houses together and he loved the work. When I got back from the meeting, he grabbed the keys, kissed my forehead, and left.

I look out the window. It's late afternoon and the pool is full of kids. The kids do backflips and cannonballs and yell, "Look Mom! Watch me, Mom!"

I feel empty. Cole bought a bunch of bananas and I eat three. I still fill empty. I dig inside my backpack for a pen.

Dear Cave Woman,

I feel empty and out of sorts.

Changing patterns will feel odd at times.

I think you've told me that before. I imagine I'll need to hear it again. I need the encouragement.

Noticing you feel odd and not immediately filling it with the promise to drink, is very encouraging. Big changes open the Survival Brain to new ways of operating.

I wish it was easier.

If recovery was easier your Survival Brain would remain on autopilot.

I need a ghost writer.

I'm your ghost writer.

Your revisions are much appreciated.

My pleasure. Your nervous system also appreciates all the revisions, which will benefit you in all areas of your life.

Am I in the 3F Red Zone less often?

Yes, the result of your own persistence. You're changing and that takes time and lots of rest.

A lot is changing, I agree, and that's good. The reasons for changing, not so good. I've always felt pressure to become someone entirely different. My father needled me from the get-go and wanted me to change and become someone else entirely. I didn't know how to do that. My mom wanted me to be myself. Sadly, I never felt relaxed enough to trust that.

Your father demanded perfection and continually reminded you of how you fell short. Demanding perfection creates relentless self-blame. A patriarchal culture seeks the upper hand by making people dependent and subservient.

But my situation wasn't that bad. I had a place to live and our family looked fine.

When it comes to abuse, no matter the reason or degree, addiction thrives.

Do all alcoholics share the same background?

All conditions vary but everyone feels the absence of

a vibrant community. **Without someone to articulate that absence, the conditions for post-traumatic stress surge.**

We're more vulnerable to PTSD without a healthy community?

Much more vulnerable. That's correct. Let's leave off the D. It's not a disorder. Post-traumatic stress is a natural response to unhealed trauma. No need to pathologize the stress that follows trauma.

Can we recover from childhood trauma?

People can recover but denying trauma can cause the PTS symptoms to linger.

For example?

For example, a little girl who is raped by her uncle could potentially find resilience in life. But if she bravely tells an adult and isn't believed, she's left without safe people to help her heal.

Damn, patriarchy has this system rigged. What should she have done?

Her impulse will always lead her to seek someone who will believe her, but her socialization will push her to stay silent. We always root for finding a safe person.

Did losing healthy communities embolden predators and isolate victims?

Tragically, yes. When we tell someone our truth and that person doesn't believe us, it leads us to question our own perceptions, even when we know exactly what happened. Then victims blame themselves and think they're defective. They may act out or they may act completely out of character or develop addictions. Instead of receiving help, they get rejected and further confirmation they're somehow defective.

Because our difficulties are judged as our fault, and we're called crazy?

That's correct. Modern humans aren't able to articulate the absence they feel. No one ever sat you down, until now, and explained why you might feel so lost, unmoored, and rebellious. No one ever explained why you were searching for a fix.

What are the symptoms of PTS?

The ones you will be most familiar with are insomnia, obsessively replaying events, practicing future conversations, unrelenting self-blame, experiencing repetitive physical reactions to thoughts or situations, and, of course, addiction.

So, PTS and a chronic 3F Red Zone are linked?

Very much so.

What about flashbacks? I don't have flashbacks.

Yes, you do. Remember you have emotional flashbacks?

A flashback with no visuals?

That's right, no strong images.

Are there other symptoms of PTS?

Symptoms reflect the ways your Survival Brain stays in protection mode, often overriding your ability to make choices or decisions.

Like what sensations specifically, for me?

Other sensations you may recall are feeling like you're not in your body, clumsiness, a short fuse, headaches, an insistent need to get away, an underlying annoyance or despair, hypervigilance. Again, you'll recognize these from chronically entering the 3F Red Zone.

I understand why I felt stuck in addiction, without hope, for so long.

Addiction steals hope and instead creates the illusion the addictive substance is the only way to regain hope. Reengage with your whole hive and you'll find hope to spare.

I remember in junior high school, a former junky gave a speech. I may have been in seventh grade, I'm not sure. I think he meant to scare us about the dangers of drugs, but as he described the ecstasy he felt during his first fix, my mouth watered. My arms longed for the prick of a needle. I never did shoot up, but afterwards I sought out the girls in the bathroom smoking pot and started going to parties to get high and drink.

The ex-junky who spoke at your school talked about how he filled the void but not why a void existed in the first place.

That stupid "Just Say No" campaign.

Explaining the dangers of drugs and alcohol rarely deters people. Learning why drugs are captivating from the start can prevent use or abuse.

Longing for a healthy community is the original craving?

That's right.

Being told our experience is not our experience causes post-traumatic stress?

Right again. With help, you could have overcome the abuse you suffered, but others' ignorance and denial left you exposed.

But my mom loved me?

Your mom loved you tremendously.

How did I wind up with PTS if I got so much love?

The Survival Brain highlights danger above all else.

And I was searching for safety?

You were searching for the safety of an encircling community.

Which is what I found in drinking?

Yes, and the rituals of the ragtag community that came with drinking.

I rarely see any of my family because they only know me through the critical eyes of my father. But a few years ago, my sister paid me a surprise visit. She'd been going through a divorce and living with our dad temporarily. During a tour of the local scenery, she said, "Living with Dad again has not been easy. I guess it never was. He was tough on me, but I can see now that you had it worst of all."

"Is he still making me out to be the devil himself?" I asked.

"He's like a dog with a bone. He takes zero responsibility for anything and blames you for everything. Even when his car needs gas, he blames you. I didn't see it before. Living with him as an adult, I see it all the time."

"I appreciate that more than I can say." I thought I might cry because I felt a little glint of hope that day.

Your sister gave you one of the most precious gifts your people can receive; validation of your perception and the knowledge that you could trust your own knowing. There are a few good healers in your world who could have provided that validation. Your sister helped launch you into recovery that day.

—◊—

Pot Stickers

Odell invited me to lunch with several women who attended her potluck supper. We're meeting at a Chinese restaurant in a strip mall about twenty minutes from my hotel. I follow the GPS directions and wonder how anyone got around without an electronic voice leading the way. The voice seems to get increasingly annoyed with me each time she tells me to turn around and I don't obey fast enough. Or maybe I'm electropomorphizing.

At the restaurant, each table has a lazy Susan in the center that spins to share family-style dishes. We start with several platters filled with pot stickers.

Charlotte, who takes care of her elderly mother, gives us a run-down on both of their ailments. It's a long list and I eat four pot stickers before I remember to make sure there are enough for everyone. There are six of us and four plates with eight pot stickers per plate. That's thirty-two pot stickers total. That leaves about five pot stickers each. I can safely have one more. I usually need paper and pen, even for simple equations. Bless my brain for working a bit better today. Bless the person who formed each one of these bits of doughy perfection.

Jane is hosting the monthly potluck supper next month and asks if I'd like to attend. I say, "Yes, thank you. I would like that." I look down and frown, wondering if I can handle one more outing, sober.

Jane asks, "Are you okay?"

I look up and say, "I'm sorry. I was just wondering if sobriety gets easier. I mean being around people in the evening. Without drinking. Does that get easier?"

She smiles and offers to pour me some tea. I nod yes. She says, "Yes and no. If drinking was the only way you could tolerate an event or if drinking was the only reason to go, those things will fall away. Or you'll make a quick appearance and leave. But yes, in general, staying sober gets much easier."

She gives me a kind smile that reminds me of my mom and heavy tears fall toward the teacup in my hands. "I'm sorry," I say. "Crying happens all the time and I don't know why."

Everyone laughs at me again.

I look up and blubber, "I'm a freak."

They laugh even harder and I'm missing the joke.

A muscular woman named Rosa, with soft brown skin and a black-and-white striped jumpsuit, says, "I cried every day for the first six months of my recovery. I cried at meetings, on the phone with every woman at this table…plus many more. I cried at my desk. Thank goodness for those awful cubical walls. I told my colleagues I had terrible allergies. It's funny to me now but at the time, I really did think I might drown in all those tears."

"I cried for a solid year," says Charlotte.

"I cried a lot, too," says Marian, a woman with a bouquet of red hair coiled like a telephone cord.

"I win this one," Jane says. "I cried while reading verdicts from the bench. The courtroom thought I was really moved by the law." She bursts out laughing and we all laugh, even me.

The waiters bring more food and even though I'm no longer hungry, I eat with enthusiasm. I don't feel like a freak. I don't feel so alone. I think life could be good.

Chapter 13

Defiance

On my way back to the hotel, I notice a used bookstore and pull in. Inside, I find a roped off café at the back of the bookstore. A sign says the café is only open for breakfast.

The owner walks up beside me and introduces herself. She says I'm welcome to sit at a table and apologizes for being out of cinnamon buns.

"A friend of mine makes them and makes more and more each week but they sell out quickly. Otherwise, I run a one-woman show and can't watch the register up front and the little café here at the same time. As soon as we sell the last cinnamon bun, I close the café." She takes a breath and adds, "Did you come here hoping for a cinnamon bun?"

"No, I just had lunch with friends," I brag, "but I'll come back earlier next time."

"I hope you do. I like to talk, and you seem like a good listener," she adds and talks for ten more minutes until a customer wants to buy a book.

"Have a seat in the café. Sorry to talk so much. Come back anytime."

"I will, thank you. By the way, I like to listen to you talk." Damn, I made another friend. I text Cole to see if he needs the car. He's taking a walk and doesn't need it now. I sit down and find my notebook.

—∞—

Dear Cave Woman,

I had lunch with friends today. I wasn't perfect, but it felt good anyway. I actually cried into a cup of tea and I'm not ashamed. It might be a day for miracles. I want to be part of this community of sober women. After lunch, I worried I talked too much about myself, revealed too much. I worried I'd thrown them the broken pieces of my life with the hope they can put me back together. I'm afraid I scared them off.

I have an idea. Tell me more about your life. You and I can put some pieces together. Then you'll be a better listener and you might have some insights to share with others. Let's start with when you first meet Cole.

—∞—

I met Cole in Montana while on vacation from NYC and ended up staying. In the winter, we lived in my family's small log home near Yellowstone Park. As a kid, I thought my pioneer ancestors hewed the family homestead out of the pine forest. But in truth, it was built by my great-grandfather as a summer vacation home. My great-grandparents were sent to Montana from Salt Lake City to spread Mormonism. My parents were Jack Mormons, a term that means they'd unofficially left the church. With the Mormon church, you're either all in or all out. My brother was friends with a cousin who tied him to the church.

The cabin wasn't built for cold weather. One winter day, Cole and I nursed hangovers in the loft where the heat from the wood stove gathered.

My mom called, sounding uncharacteristically nervous, and said, "Your sister's been in therapy and the therapist wondered why we'd moved from Montana to DC right after you were born. The therapist said families just don't pick up and move two thousand miles without a good reason. She's right, and I need to tell you the real reason."

When I was six months old, my family moved across the country when my dad got a job with the federal government.

"The truth is your father was having an affair with his secretary," my mom said. She spoke rapidly and sounded winded.

"Why am I not surprised?" I said unhelpfully.

"I was pregnant with you and had two children under ten. I found him a job with the federal government, and we moved."

"I'm so sorry, Mom."

"He wants to send you $500 a month to help support you."

"Wait, he what––?" A muffled sound interrupted our conversation. Maybe she dropped the phone and couldn't get ahold of it again.

I knew she wanted to hang up the phone, which was unusual. We talked nearly every day and there were only a few topics off limits, like how her alcoholic father treated her as a child. She'd only say that he was a mean drunk. When her parents left during the Great Depression, she got a job cooking at a boarding house in exchange for a room.

I told Cole about the call and we laughed awkwardly about the money and how odd it seemed. My dad had never been fond of me. I angered and annoyed him no matter if I did well or got in trouble. I couldn't win. Now I knew why.

Dear Cave Woman,

Did I ruin my dad's life? Was I at fault for how he treated me? **He projected blame for his behavior on to you. He trained**

everyone in your family, including you, to instantly lay fault at your feet, which is what you're doing right now.

Where blame goes, addiction follows?

In the closed system you call families, yes. The children who receive blame often learn to blame themselves, especially when another sibling receives all the praise. Those who are blamed feel guilt and pressure. Yet another reason my community raised children communally. We would never risk a child feeling poorly about themselves. Our cohesiveness depended on our mutual appreciation and cooperation.

Cave woman?

Yes?

I'm tired. I'll go and lay down at the hotel.

Of course. Go rest, my sleepy sloth.

—⟪⟫—

Domino Effect

Back at the hotel, I try to nap, but instead my mind buzzes. After dinner with Cole, we watch TV and go to bed. I fall asleep while listening to an audio book. I wake up a few hours later to a quiet and still hotel room. My heart pounds with panic and I don't know why. I repeatedly change positions trying to get comfortable. I'm relieved Cole sleeps through my nightly ups and downs. I take a few Spare Tire Breaths and ask myself if this is an emotional flashback. My panic eases and I take that as a yes.

I woke up so many times with a hangover, diving straight into self-derision. I guess that's still a habit. The memories still reverberate. The panic makes sense. I use the bathroom, then get some cold water and drink deeply. I roll the cold bottle on my forehead. I still feel some fear, but I tell the fear I'm ready to listen.

Without the panic, I could learn to love the nighttime.

—⁕—

Dear Cave Woman,

Where were we?

Appreciation and cooperation.

Oh, yeah. When my mom and I were alone, we appreciated and enjoyed each other's company. A life filled with her love is more than I can imagine. No, wait. I can imagine it, through you. I love your world. I love Cole. I love my new friends.

You can imagine it because you've been finding traces of your own natural wellbeing. You enjoy learning and you're beginning to trust you can work with whatever comes up.

Should we start a commune?

No, absolutely not. When people start communes, they mistakenly bring unquestioned societal norms.

For example?

For example, the women still cook, clean, and raise babies, and the men fix cars and mow the lawn. There's no gender balance or social parity.

And they bring addictions and control issues?

Absolutely. They bring the society they're attempting to escape right along with them. Everyone brings their own idea of the perfect commune and the infighting becomes atrocious.

Are there people who are addicted to perfection?

Perfectionism can be a form of control and a source for addiction. Many people attempt to make everything and every-

one around them perfect. This is a tragic mindset since there's no such thing as human-controlled perfection. Perfectionists cause the people around them to suffer feelings of banishment.

Why do they stay if they feel rejected?

Because they're taught to believe everything is their fault. If they attempt to step back from a controlling relationship— any type of relationship—they're berated for overreacting or for being unreasonable.

I think religious guilt is used as means of control. That damn religious guilt filters into everything.

When people can't shift out of forced guilt, they blame themselves. Instead, they can question where the guilt feelings originated. Modern society loves to blame individuals for systemic problems.

But aren't control freaks rewarded with praise and adulation?

They can be, which encourages them to seek more control. When the control addict receives praise, the people around them feel invisible, rejected, and guilty.

I understand that trio. Invisibility, rejection, and guilt is a confusing combination.

And rife for self-condemnation.

What a brutal setup. Why do some people want to control so badly?

Many people are following what they learned under patriarchy; to break others' self-worth, divide people against each other, deflect blame, and maintain their own façade of perfection.

Oh, that's how control addicts make their victims seem like the crazy one?

Yes, you have a sharp eye for spotting control addicts. That's a good skill to have in the modern world.

If I listen to my first instinct.

Precisely my point.

I think—

Let's step back for a minute. I need to point out an important distinction.

There's a difference between control addicts and people who are narcissists, psychopaths, or sociopaths. The later type has no conscience and lacks empathy for anyone other than themselves. Most narcissists, psychopaths, and sociopaths are also control addicts. I'm not sure what to call them. "Narcissists, psychopaths, and sociopaths" is a mouthful.

We could make up a word?

Oh, let's. I don't know how you keep from making up words every day.

Ridicule mostly. Dreary people irritatingly say, "That's not a real word." Linguistic killjoys.

Fortunately for us, all words were made up at some point. Let's have some fun.

The word needs to mean "without empathy or without a conscience," correct?

Yes, the word will most likely be a portmanteau; a combination of two or three words. There are so many languages to choose from. What's your favorite language?

I don't know any other languages, so I don't know.

Fair enough. Let me think…what is your favorite part of the world?

Sadly, I haven't traveled much, but I'm going to the Caribbean soon.

Okay, the Caribbean. Besides English, we have German, Creole, Spanish, and Dutch, but let's see if we can keep the word short. Let me take a closer look at Creole. Here's a pos-

sibility. Haitian Creole is an engaging blend of languages. Let me think. As I investigate Haitian Creole I find "san" for without and "ke" for conscience. San-ke. What do you think of the word sanke?

Sanke—without conscience. I like it very much. Can we make up more words?

We can, but right now let's keep our focus. I know talking about sankes can be painful, but it will help you understand parts of your life that've left you baffled.

I do feel worried, but you make the night less lonely and I'm wide awake. I'd like to keep going.

Good. I'll be quick. Sankes make others feel crazy and off balance by lying habitually, even lying about inconsequential things, to keep the playing field perpetually unstable.

Sankes know how to lie and manipulate so people feel sorry for them.

Sankes deflect guilt onto their victims.

Sankes make others responsible for the sanke's happiness. By design, targets of sankes carry a heavy burden for not being good enough to make the sanke happy. Sankes are effective at manipulating people because compassion and scruples don't cloud their thought process. Empathy is not a distraction.

Sankes have no conscience, but they can act like a person with integrity as it suits their objectives.

Sankes exploit compassion to garner pity. If sankes had a currency, it would be self-pity.

Sankes always have a bigger and better tale of woe.

This all sounds very familiar. Do people like this exist because we lost our healthy communities?

No, they've always existed, they just weren't in leadership roles. In my community, we could tell at a very young age if a child lacked empathy. Some, of course, had physical conditions that we would treat and help them heal. But children born without a conscience would kill animals and hurt other children with no moral discernment or regret. They were calculating liars and carried no remorse. Sankes learned to manipulate and use others early in life.

Did you chop off their heads?

No, although that was often discussed. We trained sankes for specific tasks. They were separated from day-to-day activities and only had contact with a few people who understood their dangerous frame of mind. They were given rigorous training to keep them occupied. We trained sankes in our form of martial arts, as fighters, and as hunters for dangerous situations.

Why would you turn people who had no conscience into expert killers?

Good question. Sankes required an elevated status and constant praise and we needed to keep everyone else safe. They needed to kill and occasionally we needed meat. At times, we needed protection from sanke-led invaders. We thought we could control sankes, and they often died young because of their aggression. But eventually they seized more and more control through terror and manipulation and shattered healthy alliances.

They became the early conquerors and despots?

Yes, sankes craved more control and violently broke our communal system. Sankes dominated and coerced people into abdicating their freedom and communities in exchange for a false sense of protection.

Like mobsters?

A lot like mobsters, yes. It's difficult for non-sankes to believe the conniving malice of sankes. Once sankes took control, a domino effect occurred spreading brutality throughout the world, especially where healthy communities still existed.

Because a healthy community was a threat to their control?

The greatest threat of all.

How does this tie into addiction?

Sankes know that without a healthy community, people are vulnerable to subjugation. Treating someone as worthless leaves them searching for other ways to feel better.

And the children of sankes?

Control addicts and sankes shift the blame for their shortcomings onto their children who begin to self-blame and self-shame. It's a terrible betrayal when a sanke blames a child for a family's hardships. The children of sankes often become controlling and/or addicted.

They become addicts to blunt the betrayal?

When an adult repeatedly convinces a child that their perceptions are faulty, that child learns not to trust their own impressions. That dissonance causes the Survival Brain to generate protective patterns. The effect on a child varies.

And sankes seem just like everyone else because they know how to act the part?

Yes, and often the only way you can spot a sanke is by the damage they leave in their wake, or by your gut sense.

What kind of damage? Can you give me an example?

For example, in your family, your father praised and encouraged one child, treated one with indifference, and derided and complained about you. It was very divisive. Guess who ended up with the addiction?

I feel like a science experiment on how to make someone an alcoholic. I felt steeped in worthlessness and now I understand why. I was targeted. I was the scapegoat. It's painful to know, but also a relief. I think I might be sick.

I know it's a bittersweet realization, but I'm glad you now know to stop judging yourself so harshly.

I'm glad to know too, but not judging myself might be a tough habit to break. I always knew something was wrong, but I couldn't put my finger on it. I remember creating my own set of rules when I was a kid. I had to avoid cracks in the stone sidewalk that lined our backyard. I developed a superstition that washcloths were bad luck, and I had to go up the stairs two at a time and run down the stairs quickly. I don't remember what I thought would happen if I left the house without taking a shower, but I'd never risk it. I wore guilt like a porcupine wears quills.

You developed patterns to protect yourself from your dad's unpredictable and energy-draining behavior. You saw his misogyny echoed in the larger world.

Totally. Even rock 'n roll lyrics are filled with hatred toward women. What else?

You didn't know how to shift the shame and blame that got dumped on you, so you adopted compulsive behaviors instead. Your helpful Dividing Mind created rules that gave you a sense of stability because they were achievable. Every child needs achievable goals and helpful feedback.

It's important to note that you knew something was wrong. Your instincts were accurate.

—⚊—

I stand up and stretch. From the mini fridge, I take out a green juice, take a sip and then add a ginger shot, shake it up, and get back to Cave Woman. I'm awake but not panicky, just a bit nauseous. The ginger will help in no time.

—⟋⟍⟋—

Dear Cave Woman,

What're the different ways people fight emotions? I feel like a tabloid reporter looking for some gore, but I'm curious.

I welcome your enthusiasm and curiosity. Curiosity is very good for you. It's good for the world. Enthusiasm keeps curiosity alive.

Now back to your question. Many people stave off emotions by controlling things like money, information, and possessions. As we've discussed, some work at controlling other people. Some stave off emotions through consuming substances, shopping, or hoarding. Some stay busy all the time, or distracted, or create dramas and throw themselves in the middle and play the victim. Some only get relief from emotions when they hurt others.

Modern people sure aren't very skillful at being human.

If humans don't cultivate cooperation, ease internal and external pressure, and evolve their emotional intelligence, humankind will cease to exist.

Let me tell you a story.

One mild spring day, I was playing with other children by a stream. We'd created a town made with sticks and mud and channeled the water through tiny canals dug with a pointy stone. Spirited birds sang loudly. Occasionally, a bird would land and scamper toward the stream for a sip of water. New buds and tiny bright green grasses inspired us to build and create something new.

A woman who'd recently married into our tribe came to wash some vegetables. We were fascinated by her but tried not to stare. We greeted her shyly. The woman nodded her head, bent down by the stream, and washed the vegetables.

In our bashfulness, we awkwardly bumped into each other. As we worked, one of us stepped on a stick lodged under a mud house and quick as lightning, mud flew straight into that poor woman's head.

She was on us in an instant and began slapping our heads and our bare arms. We were stunned. We'd never seen an adult hit a child before and were as shocked as if we'd seen a mouse give birth to a fish. I cried and wanted to get away.

As we ran away, she yelled that we better not tell anyone. We stopped and looked at the ground and at each other. We were taught that secrets can be very dangerous. We shared our nudges and knowledge. Even the smallest detail can be a vital clue to impending danger. We'd all told lies hoping for an extra treat or wanting to look good, but this felt precarious. We shrugged and nodded and went home with rocks in our stomachs.

But a glum lot of children on a spring day was too unusual not to garner attention.

It didn't take much prodding until we spilled the beans.

When the woman returned, she gave us each a mean look that stung almost as much as being hit.

That night at the fire, the adults shared stories of getting into trouble as children. I laughed until my belly hurt at the stories of their misdeeds. It occurred to me for the first time they'd been children too and I loved them even more. No one mentioned hitting or that it was peculiar to us. But It didn't take long before the new woman started laughing just as hard as the rest of us.

Dear Cave Woman,

You taught her that humiliation was not how you disciplined children without humiliating her.

Precisely. Humiliating her would not have helped make our case. Just the opposite. Humiliating her would have been like a slap in the face and perpetuated the physical and emotional abuse. No one's life was in immediate danger, so we had the luxury of teaching and learning as if we had all the time in the world.

Chapter 14

Paradoxical Pairs of Opposites

Dear Cave Woman,

It's near dawn, and I need to confess a fear. I don't want to talk about this particular fear in depth. Can I tell you and we'll just keep it light? Is that an odd request?

Not at all. I suggest you tell me the fear very briefly and instead of talking about the issue, I'll teach you a new skill to handle the fear.

Yes, please. I need another way to handle fear.

And?

And, I have a terrible feeling the job in Haiti is a bust. That's all I want to say right now.

Understood. So, when you look at your fears, you'll often find pairs of opposites.

You fear speaking up and you also fear keeping quiet.

You fear participating and you fear feeling left out.

You fear being thrown away and you fear being asked to stay.

If I have opposite fears, does that mean they're not real?

You can experience all sorts of contradictory feelings. Let's unwind this a little further. Write down your fears and then write down the opposite statement.

—◊◊◊—

I rip out a piece of paper, fold it in half, and list my fears on one side and turn it over and list the opposite statement.

—◊◊◊—

Dear Cave Woman,

Statements written. Now what?

Which statement, the fear or its opposite, feels better in your body? Can you feel how statements from the Unreliable Narrator feel heavy or yucky?

Oh, that's a good one. My body definitely tenses up when I reread certain statements. I can see the Unreliable Narrator statements. My body is an Unreliable Narrator detector. This really works.

The more familiar you become with sensations in your body, the more support you'll feel.

But I don't feel unconditional support like you did. Did you feel it even without emergency rooms, hospitals, antibiotics, or grocery stores?

Without a doubt.

My world was a living breathing emergency room for the heart and soul. We kicked up protective microorganisms with every step we took. We rarely needed antibiotics and had healing rituals and two dozen remedies if we did.

You knew what remedies would work when you were sick?

Many remedies were passed down through the generations. But we knew which plants or minerals would work because healing remedies that usually tasted bitter, tasted sweet when we were ill. As soon as they started to taste bitter, the dose was complete. Animals medicate themselves in the same manner.

Could I do that now?

Of course, if you can source good remedies.

I'll look into that. What else?

We never set ourselves apart or against each other. Above all, we didn't have to distract ourselves from life's crashing waves because we knew the waves well. We could be dashed about and still recover our equilibrium, together.

Weren't you afraid of death? Weren't the women in your tribe afraid to die in childbirth without an emergency room?

We didn't dread dying the way your people do. This gave us a freedom you haven't yet found. We saw death and birth as essentially the same thing. I might say goodbye to a beloved friend only to see her reemerge as a newborn a few days later.

How did you know it was her?

I didn't, but my love was the same. Also, without abuse, exploitation, and division, all life is just life transforming. Life, at its core, is limitless and incorruptible. The only way to interrupt unconditional support is to separate from each other in all the prejudicial and abusive ways modern people have inherited and left unquestioned.

I stand up, yawn, and stretch. The air around me is vibrating. I lightly imagine being a part of a wave and I feel exhilarated. I take a shower and let the water get nice and hot. I have a lot of fear, but now I know that some of my fears are inaccurate, thanks to my brilliant body. Knowing fear will never let me turn away from what matters most is heartening. I'm not so afraid of fear anymore.

Chapter 15

The Dance of Recovery

This morning I'm headed to another meeting. I'm a better driver when I'm not hungover and I easily find the meeting, which is in a small adobe church.

I find a seat, and when it's time to share, a woman with short black hair that highlights her light blue eyes shares first. She holds herself and struggles not to cry. "I finally spoke with my daughter today," she says with a voice hoarse from crying.

No one makes a sound in this old adobe chapel. Several church buildings surround us, newer and much larger, but I like this little one-room church with hand-hewn beams in the ceiling. The sun shines through narrow vertical windows revealing hundreds of descending dust moats.

"Five days ago, my ex told me my baby had been diagnosed with a form of cancer that's fast moving and fatal. My precious little girl is only thirteen years old and I was desperate to talk to her." She takes a sip of coffee from a paper coffee cup.

We don't comment on anyone's share so everyone feels free to speak openly. I wonder if that rule has some wiggle room and if people will console her directly. I stay silent and give her all my attention.

"I kept leaving my daughter messages on my ex's phone, but my daughter only called back this morning." Her tears flow freely now. "And she refuses to see me. She said I wasn't her mother and haven't been since I chose drinking over her and her father."

I expect gasps and a rush to her side. Instead, we continue to sit in silence, listening diligently.

"You want to know why? You want to know why my beloved dying daughter won't see me?" She practically spits out the words, "Because I couldn't put down the bottle.

"Alcoholism caused so much destruction and loss. My ex took our daughter across the country to get away from me and now she won't even see me. I told her I'd been in recovery since they left." She stops and looks out the window.

I follow her eyes and look outside, too. The reverential cacti stand like bodyguards in the church courtyard. One bows toward us slightly, listening respectfully. I imitate the cacti, lean closer and witness.

"She said it's too late. I'd never see her again. But it's just dawned on me. As I sit here, as I'm talking, I understand. She didn't have a say about a damn thing when I was drinking. She was helpless and now she's not. I get to keep saying no to drinking and she gets to say no to me. She has every right to be a powerful young woman." She smiles proudly and nods her head several times. She looks around the room with admiration. "Thank you all for being here. Thank goodness we don't have to spend the rest of our lives—however long that may be—wondering what might have been if only we'd gotten sober. We get to stand up for ourselves right now, no matter what we did in the past. We get to be who we should have been all along. On opposite sides of the country, my daughter and I get to be powerful women for once in our lives. I'm really proud of her. She's not punishing me. She's showing me that it wasn't all bad by standing her ground and being true to herself." I wait for someone to jump in and tell her that her daughter might change her mind, or everything will be okay, or to tell her that everything happens for a reason; the most cringe-worthy and invalidating comment I know.

After about a minute of elongated silence, another woman speaks. She talks about how her boss is giving her a hard time and how she fears drinking again if she doesn't find a new job.

I've never seen such a level playing field. One woman's young daughter might die, and another woman can't keep working for a rotten boss. We never know what might threaten our sobriety, what might revive our terrible thirst. Telling our stories freely, in turn, makes a world of difference. For these two women with disparate problems, addiction makes them equal partners in the dance of recovery.

After the meeting, a group surrounds the mom with the sick daughter. They seem to know each other already, so I catch up with the woman with the difficult boss and ask if she'd like to talk. We walk to her car and exchange phone numbers. She gives me more details, and I offer to help with her resume, and we both feel better.

Screwbeans

After the meeting, I sit at a picnic table next to a small stream under a screwbean tree. A helpful plaque tells me screwbeans are delicious and nutritious.

—⚉—

Dear Cave Woman,

Greif is on my mind today. I need to write something down, but it will be painful. I need you with me.

I'm with you. Eager to listen.

"A great burden has been lifted from me," my dad said when he called one early spring day to tell me my mom had died. "I'm not going to have a funeral. Since I'm having a party on the 4th of July anyway, we'll scatter her ashes then."

My stomach flinched, and my heart stilled, then let go with a thud. I'm sure many people throughout time have simultaneously felt helpless rage and grief. My arms desired a heavy sword to hurl through the phone lines and across my father's neck. I wanted to yell, "Murderer!" into the phone.

Instead, I hung up.

Nine years after my mom's fall, my brother-in-law witnessed my dad pushing his finger aggressively down her throat to make her swallow a pill. My dad forced several more pills down her throat in the same manner as she choked and cried. Through gritted teeth, he told her to shut up and hit the back of her head. It was the first time someone other than me had seen my dad physically abuse my mom. No one believed me when I'd told them about my father's physically abusive behavior. I'd contact a relative or a family friend I thought he might listen to and force him to get help. He always said I was lying and that he and my mom were fine. Or he'd lie and tell them I'd promised to care for my mom, but I hadn't shown up yet.

While visiting, I watched him manhandle dressing and feeding her and then choke and hit her when she couldn't keep up. One day, I helped her get dressed using kind direction. Mom remained relaxed and comfortable, but my dad couldn't believe I hadn't used brute force.

I said I'd quit both my jobs, leave Cole, and take care of Mom if he would take her to a neuropsychologist and follow their plan for her rehabilitation.

The doctors said she has Alzheimer's. I don't have time for that. Do you know what something like that would cost?" he said.

I don't think people get instant Alzheimer's," I said, flummoxed as always by his ease with lying and disregard for my mother's welfare.

I had no power to change his mind and only one equally powerless person who believed what was happening.

Getting my mom in a nursing home took another six months after my brother-in-law witnessed what I'd seen for years. Tragically, my dad spent all day with her at the home, continuing the abuse. I called the nursing home and told the director about my father's abuse. She said she would pretend she didn't hear me because they'd be liable, and she hung up.

The whole world seemed rigged to cover up abuse.

The images of the person I loved most in the world being mistreated replayed in my mind night and day. Heavy with helplessness, I worked a lot and drank. So, when a friend suggested building bamboo houses in Haiti as a sustainable way to provide affordable housing, I jumped on it like a cat on a mouse. Maybe all this suffering had a greater purpose.

I couldn't help my own mom, but maybe I could be useful to the world in some other way.

What a naïve fool I was.

—⋙—

I stop writing, stand, and look closely at a dangling bunch of screwbeans. They fold into each other's support. Tears fall, and I let the ground take them. I wipe my face on my sleeve and look at my notebook. I suspect I'm still a naïve fool. Cave Woman will tell me.

—⋙—

Dear Cave Woman,

I'm so worthless. I couldn't even help my own mom. What if

I'm not worthy of a new life? With this awful track record, I don't qualify for any healthy community.

Condemning yourself perpetuates helplessness, which helps no one. As your past surfaces, so do long-buried personal insights and resources within your own organism and the life source that surrounds you.

If I stop condemning myself, will I become a different person?

You'll recall your innate resources. That will feel different, more spacious and well-equipped. All humanity could benefit from recovery, in one form or another.

I have a question about something you said earlier. What's the life force that surrounds me?

What you see with your eyes is just a small part of your being. It's good to practice feeling the energy around you. As you begin to sense this vastness, many burdens you carry will move through you more easily. Instead of hanging on, they'll move like—

Like poop?

Yes, actually, a lot like digestion. You want to digest life's experiences, not let them build up inside you and cause a backup. You should energetically poop several times a day.

My thoughts and feelings are toxic?

Stagnation can cause discomfort and distort your perception. Ask yourself what helpful messages your feelings have for you?

I just asked this big lump of sadness what information it had for me, and it said, "Life is so sad." That wasn't very useful.

Perhaps ask what *helpful* information sadness has for you.

Okay. Sadness, what *helpful* information do you have for me?

And what did it say?

It said, "Hiding from the world's problems is the problem," which doesn't seem very sad.

Does "Hiding from the world's problems is the problem" make sense to you?

Yes, it does. The world and all the terrible injustice freaks me out, which paralyzes me and, as you said, helps no one. And all the sadness, over all those years, wanted me to see how I was mired in overwhelm? I'm kind of stunned.

Sadness helps us grieve and release the person we once were for who we're becoming. Sadness helps clear out the lingering residue.

Can it hurry the hell up?

You want to flip a switch and be done with the past. Instead, let sadness help you usher out old ways of thinking and reacting. Let sadness do its work.

I always hate when people say, "Just let it go." If I could just let it go, I would! Are you saying I can recover just by letting it all go?

Every time you write to me, you transmute old energy. Every day you don't consume alcohol, outdated patterns drop away. When people say, "Let it go," it can feel dismissive. I understand. I won't ever ask you to just let it go.

Thank you. Can I do this sobriety thing on my own now? I'm not sure I can handle other people's grief and sadness.

If someone hadn't shared their grief and sadness today, you wouldn't have shared yours with me.

Maybe I should stay away from people for a while. I sure seem to have a bad temper lately.

Actually, you need to spend even more time in the company of other people in recovery. They'll provide cover while you gather some resiliency and rebuild your hive.

Are they my new community?

Some of them, yes. You'll explore many avenues and find

ideas and friends from different walks of life, philosophies, healing traditions, and even other times and dimensions.

Like you?

Yes, like me. I lived in my time, and I've also watched humans throughout history. I've seen humanity take many wrong turns. Changing course requires a gutsiness to view what you call reality differently.

You and the screwbean tree are all the different I can handle right now.

—⟋⟋⟍—

Prioritize

The next day, at another meeting, I'm angry, but I'm not sure I know why. The drop ceiling in this room is far too low. Three large tables have been pushed together, and I can't position my feet without hitting a table leg. I'd like to throw the tables and chairs out the door and sit on the floor.

"My son didn't talk with me for three years after I got sober," says a manicured woman in a fitted pink dress and a diamond ring the size of a raisin. "I had to learn to trust my son to know when the time was right.

"It was excruciating, and I cried pretty much every day. In meetings. At night. On the phone with my sponsor." She retrieves a pink handkerchief from her white leather bag and continues, "If I didn't cry, the worry would creep in, and I'd start thinking about how good a drink sounded. But I had to show my son I was better, not just tell him. He'd heard it all before. The promises of how I'd never drink again, how sorry I was, how I'd get help this time. That poor kid.

"I only drank on weekends, and I thought that meant I wasn't an alcoholic. I thought I was living the good life and having a great time. I played the good mom during the week and partied on the weekends. I dreamed about drinking all week long and couldn't pour that Friday afternoon drink fast enough.

"Each time I got arrested for drunk driving, I was shocked. I never remembered leaving the house, but I remember the arrest. For some odd reason, I'd come to as soon as the siren sounded. I don't understand why they had to be so rough with me, though. But I guess I could have killed someone or myself. I'm not a criminal, and police officers need to learn we have a problem. I still think it's unfair."

I was pretty sure she had committed a crime by driving drunk, and the Black women in the room probably could tell her about being pulled over unfairly.

One of the Black women introduces herself. Her library glasses, her ironed linen shorts, and Hawaiian shirt highlight her casual elegance. Uh-oh, I think the woman in pink is about to get schooled.

"I can so relate to your story. Thank you for being honest. I know being honest about what it was like—the unvarnished truth—is what keeps me sober and what finally got my kids to tentatively start trusting me again.

"My kids were seven, nine, and ten when I finally got sober this last time. I was so ashamed, but my counselor told me that if I held on to the shame, it would take me back to the bottle. It was the best advice I'd ever received. I tell the truth whenever I feel shame and let the chips fall where they may. Sobriety is my number one priority, and she demands complete honesty."

She looked me right in the eye and flashed a brief smile. I smiled back. I like the idea of consulting my recovery like she's a goddess or a genie.

She continued, "My kids and I are closer than ever, and I owe my life to the women in this room and all the women in all the rooms like it. My counselor told me something else that changed my life. She said that my mother's suicide significantly increased the chances of taking my own life. Suicide could potentially seem like a solution to me because it was the only solution my mother could find. Just like alcohol was my solution to every problem, suicide, for my mother, was her solution.

"I knew I had to make the conscious decision that I would not pass on alcohol as a solution to my kids. I knew I had to learn not to think about suicide as a solution, either. We talk about addiction and suicide, which are some of the most powerful conversations we've ever had. Talking about solutions that work, sometimes over days and weeks, makes all the difference in how close we are today. Thank you all for being here. I couldn't do it without you."

The next woman speaks, and I'm horrified to find it's me. After I begin talking, I stumble. I had an idea about what to say but it's gone, so I say, "I just wanted to introduce myself. I was told to just listen but I don't know…I just…you know…I just kinda like the idea that these meetings aren't the answer but it's how we find the answer… you know, solutions. Oh, crap. I should be quiet…that doesn't even make sense…anyway, I'm Sil, and I belong here. Obviously." I expected to speak elegantly like the woman who had spoken before me, a woman who had many years of sobriety behind her. What was I thinking? Why couldn't I just keep my mouth shut? My heart beats in my throat so insistently it feels like I am riding a trotting elephant.

As the meeting ends, I'm mad at the woman in pink for saying the police were unfair to pull her over while driving drunk. I'm surprised to see the Black woman leave without talking to her. The only two people left in the room are the woman in pink and me. That is when it hits me. I'm the one who needs to say something.

"Excuse me," I say, "I wanted to ask about something you said. You said you thought it was unfair to be pulled over, but do you know Black people get pulled over all the time just because they're Black?"

Her straight back slumps, and she sighs, "I do know that. Thank you for saying something. I'll make some phone calls and apologize to the group next time. I can be so thoughtless."

"We all need reminders," I say and quickly add, "I need reminders."

"We'll remind each other. Would you like to join me for a cup of coffee?" she asks.

I surprise myself and say, "Okay, let's meet at the corner café."

At the café, we play a game. We think of all the things we think we know and all the ways we forget daily. And how we take so much for granted, what we prioritize, and how we could each put more effort into educating ourselves.

I say, "They keep telling us in meetings we'll learn to be less selfish and be of service to others...."

"What a good reminder. I seem to conveniently forget about the service to others part. What's the point otherwise? When I was in law school, I wanted to be a civil rights lawyer. I've become so selfish. I can get back on track. Thanks for helping me remember." She adds, "This has been an illuminating conversation for me."

"Illuminating for us both," I add.

Madeline

Heading toward the hotel, a car stops beside me at a traffic light. A cat peeks over the window and stares at me. She looks so much like Maddy. The elephant stampedes through my heart again, and a sign for a liquor store catches my eye. I put on my blinker and turn in. I

park and reach for my backpack and feel my notebook inside. I sink
back in my seat. Damnit, Cave Woman. I root around for my pen.

—◊◊◊—

Dear Cave Woman,

Recovery is impossible. I'll always think about leaving Maddy
and hate myself. Hating myself gives me the terrible thirst.

Besides, cravings are so unpredictable and impossible to catch
before it's too late.

**Actually, you just caught a craving. Check yourself and
you'll see that it's gone.**

What did you do?

**I was just here. You thought about Maddy and felt bad,
and you wanted it to stop.**

I feel such brutal remorse. I'm having trouble catching my breath.
I'll never stay sober if I keep feeling this way. What should I do?

Do you love her?

Of course.

Then do that.

You make it sound so easy.

We can unwind what just happened if that'll help.

Okay, good. I'd like to unwind.

**Write about how you ended up in the parking lot of a
liquor store and what stopped you from going inside.**

As I grabbed my backpack to buy wine, I remembered what
you said about suppressing emotions with alcohol. I saw a cat like
the one I'd given away, and regret rushed through me. The regret
didn't drive my car into the parking lot. It was just an old habitual
response to curb unpleasant feelings. Is that right?

Very good.

The regret is profound. My chest feels like it's being squeezed like King Kong has me in his grip high above Manhattan. I'm afraid to look down. Oh, gawd, I looked down and there's a lot of fear here. Now the elephant has one leg on my stomach.

Is the elephant leaning its full weight against your stomach?

When I think about an actual elephant, I'd have to say it's just touching my stomach.

Now it feels like a squirrel is running around inside my chest. Boy, that's unpleasant.

Are you contracting any muscles?

Oh, yeah. It's like my pelvic muscles and my shoulder muscles are conspiring to fold me in half.

That's how they protect your organs from sharp tusks. Are you breathing from your chest?

Oh, right. Spare Tire breathing. Okay, got it. I need another break.

Take all the breaks you need.

—⟋⟍—

I sit up a little straighter and take three Spare Tire Breaths. My mind whirls with thoughts of telling Maddy how sorry I am. I wish more than anything I'd never left Maddy. The panic in my chest feels like an electrical short. I put the window down, and I ask Maddy if she'd known my betrayal would be the reason I finally got sober. I take three more Spare Tire Breaths and lean against the headrest. A truck rumbles by loudly playing, "We Are The Champions." I smile as tears fall along my cheeks.

—⟋⟍—

Dear Cave Woman,

I'm back. I doubt I'll ever feel guilt-free about leaving Maddy.

I betrayed her. I also have this strange feeling she can feel how I feel, and my need to wallow in guilt is not helping her. Or am I making that up just to feel better?

Does it matter? Tell me, what would drinking accomplish?

Drinking would only continue the betrayal. I think I'll write to Maddy and thank her for helping me get sober. Can you stay with me?

I'll be here when you need me. Good job recognizing a Yellow Caution Zone before you slid into red.

I can't find a comfortable position, and my joints start aching. I feel a burning in my right shoulder and then in my hips and knees. Now my wrists and elbow burn, too. I struggle to take in enough oxygen. The pain remains, but I don't care.

I heard from the no-kill shelter today where Cole and I left Maddy. She was adopted by a family with a big fancy mansion. Their last cat was a tortoiseshell like Maddy. There's no going back. I'll never see her again. My mind wasn't working well when I left her to try and save the world. I should have taken care of her. I should have gotten help. I talked Cole into this whole crazy trip.

Honestly, I couldn't bear grieving my mom and instead made more hurt in the world.

Right now, I just want to go beg the people who adopted her to let me take her back. I want to beg Maddy to give me another chance to care for her. It seems like the only thing that will ease the pain.

Instead, I write pages and pages, and then I rip them up. No amount of words can adequately express my regret. Regret is such a paltry word to describe such a massive black hole. I make a list of why I'm the worst person in the world and a list of as many regrets as I can remember.

It is an awfully long list.

I crumple each piece of paper into a tight ball and find a paper sack in the backseat. I fill up the bag, and I scrunch it up enough to grip the top. The closest trash can is near the liquor store entrance, which no longer tempts me. I stuff the bag in and imagine the pages consumed by fire until there's nothing left, not even a smudge of ash. As I walk back toward the car, I flip off the bottles of wine glistening behind me, whispering curse words with each step.

I call Odell and tell her how I ended up in a liquor store parking lot. I cry and wipe my nose on my shirt and tell her about what I wrote.

She listens and then asks if I can drive back to the hotel without stopping at another liquor store. I say yes, and we hang up.

I have to buy some tissues for my car. I put the car in gear and slowly drive back to the hotel. Fortunately, I've started wearing a swimsuit under my clothes. I take off my black cotton pants and purple long-sleeve T-shirt, throw them on a lounge chair, and take a quick swim. If Cole asks why my eyes are so red, I'll blame the chlorine.

Bootleg

Cole isn't fooled by my chlorine excuse and asks why I'd been crying.

I accidentally blurt out the truth before I can wonder if It'll upset him. "I feel so awful about leaving Maddy, but I think that's why I'm in recovery. Does that make any sense at all?" I beg.

"Not really," Cole says kindly as he puts his strong arms around me in a hug.

I hug him back and say again, "I just feel really awful."

"I know. I do too."

I cry and get his shirt wet. "I made a mess of things and hurt you and Maddy because I couldn't grieve what happened to my mom. How can you even stand to be around me?"

"I have an idea. How about we share the guilt? I was there too, remember? We made a choice together. Now, you're getting help and that matters to me."

"I'm gonna have to spend the rest of my life making this up to her."

"I'll help. Okay? Are you hungry?"

We order a pizza and watch TV before we go to bed.

I thought I might sleep tonight after all those tears but no luck. I'm not at all sleepy. I feel like I have the outside edges of a puzzle done, but the middle pieces are missing.

—◊—

Dear Cave Woman,

I've been told all my life I'm too sensitive.

By whom?

My dad and all the people he constantly tells I'm too sensitive. By the culture all around me. By people who undervalued my work and labor and don't pay well. By a world that is sensitive-phobic.

Sensitivity is a gift in your world. Sensitivity requires a lot of strength without the support of a wise, continuous community.

That makes no sense at all. How on Earth is sensitivity a gift? How can I be strong and sensitive? I'm so sensitive I dropped out of school in sixth grade because of a stupid bully.

You dropped out of school because you already had a bully at home. Tell me about when you dropped out of school. Then tell me a fond memory you have of your mom.

Okay, I'll tell you a story for a change.

——ɷ——

From the school bus, I saw Ada's older brother chasing her around a sloped yard next to their narrow weather-beaten house. The exhaust from the idling bus made me feel sick. Ada's brother pushed her against an old misshapen oak tree and slugged her a few times before taunting her about being late for school. He said the word school like it was a bad thing, and that part I understood.

I had my mom to myself during the day. School took that away, and each day felt endless. I wished I could be like the people in movies who loved school so much they won awards and became brilliant scientists and explorers. I couldn't imagine what school they went to, but it couldn't possibly be any I'd attended, and I'd been to several. We lived on the edge of two school districts, and I tried going back and forth between different schools.

I liked one teacher. She was older than most of the other teachers, had short hair, and always wore jeans and a denim shirt. She helped us plant trees on Earth Day in early spring and taught us about the medicinal properties of plants. Then, one day she got a job in the principal's office. I'd see her inside the hushed glassed-in office, away from the roar of students changing classes, and wish she'd stayed a teacher.

Shop class was fun with the slightly burnt smell of freshly cut pine. I liked how the saw blades sliced through wood with such precision. I enjoyed making a mess with sawdust and wood scraps and taking something home besides boring textbooks. I loved to read, but my textbooks were as heavy as they were boring. I'd promise myself each week to do all my assignments but would end up falling asleep at my modern new desk, bought just so I could study better. My mind would wander a hundred times until I gave up and picked up a library book from the pile by my bed.

The swoosh and clunk of the school bus door closing brought my attention back to Ada.

As she walked to her seat, everyone looked at the floor. I looked her right in the eye to let her know I understood. My siblings hadn't hit me, but my dad had.

Instead, she looked at me with such scorn that I knew I was next.

I crossed my arms and slumped down in my seat. The bus moved, the exhaust cleared, and a hit of adrenaline chased my nausea away. By the time I got to my locker, she'd rounded up some friends to hold me while she gut-punched me until the bell rang.

I didn't tell anyone at school. I told my mom, and I refused to return. I dropped out of school in sixth grade. Being home with my mom was so much better. She ironed, which smelled like pancakes cooking in a cast-iron skillet, while we watched old movies and I learned the history of film. At least the ones that played on channel 31 out of Baltimore. We folded laundry in the dark hallway so we could see the sparks—like a meteor shower in the night sky—as my mom peeled the clothes apart. I learned about static electricity, and we talked about lightning. We added books about clouds, astronomy, and film history to our list for the library.

One early spring morning, my mom said she wanted to show me something outside. A tall tulip poplar tree spanned the side of the house and held the shade and humidity. Jungle-like plants and bright green moss covered the ground. My mom crouched at the base of the tree and pointed toward a jack-in-the-pulpit. The proud stamen was covered by a protective leaf but still held a view of the world like a spyglass from Mother Earth herself. My mouth hung open in wonder.

I kept looking between my mom and the jack-in-the-pulpit, wondering if this might be my initiation into a magical realm like Narnia or Camelot. My mom always said magic was everywhere. I was beginning to understand.

We made a game of everything. She gathered things that needed to be put away in a big paper sack and had me reach in and identify them by feel. When I guessed correctly, I "won" by getting to put it away. She taught me what it meant to "Huck Fin" someone, which meant tricking someone into doing something you'd rather not do yourself. We put Huckleberry Fin on the library list, too.

Toward the end of the day, my anxiety would bubble up as my dad and siblings began arriving home. I'd ask my mom for one of her stories to quell the quiver in my stomach.

She and her best friend Rita got into the best trouble.

"Did I ever tell you Rita and I used to bootleg whiskey?"

"No way," I said. I was so impressed I jumped up and almost overturned my chair.

She smiled wide, ate a bit of a carrot, and continued, "This wasn't during prohibition. That ended when I was little. This was during the Second World War. Liquor was rationed, and each state was allotted only so many bottles."

I sat at the kitchen table as Mom washed and cut up broccoli for a casserole. It smelled skunky, but I knew it would be deliciously drowned in lots of creamy cheese sauce.

"I was living at Rita's house most of the time. Her stepdad owned a bar downtown."

"How old were you?"

She handed me the grater and a block of cheddar cheese. I was a slow grater.

Mom moved on to washing and patting the chicken dry. "I think we would have been about twelve or thirteen. I'm not sure where Rita's mom was, but we were on our own a lot." She sautéed the chicken in butter with mushrooms, onions, and a splash of white wine.

I wished dinner was ready, and I ate some cheese to ease the hunger. "Do you know why?" I asked.

"I guess they trusted us or, more likely, they were living it up because of the war, like a lot of people. It seemed like a lot of kids were on their own."

I looked outside and couldn't imagine our suburban neighborhood without parents imposing arbitrary rules and ruining flashlight tag.

"Each bottle had a sticker put on by the state so it couldn't be sold in a different state. We'd scrape off the Utah stickers with razor blades, and then we'd put on the Montana stickers."

"Where did you get the Montana stickers?"

"The sheriff," Mom said as she slid the casserole in the oven.

"No way. The sheriff?" I said, enjoyably shocked.

"Rita's stepdad bought them from the sheriff. One time Rita and I had to meet the sheriff in front of the house and give him the envelope of money for the stickers. Rita's stepdad had already left to open the bar. We were scared out of our wits. The sheriff asked us, 'You girls aren't going to tell anyone about this, are you?' Without missing a beat, Rita said, 'No sir, we have to make a living, too.' Something she'd heard her stepdad say dozens of times. The sheriff was still laughing when his police car turned the corner a block down the street."

"Then what?" I asked.

"To get the stickers to stay in place, we put the bottles in the oven. Of course, we had to be careful they didn't get too hot. We opened the oven so many times to check, I'm surprised any of them stuck at all. Then when Rita's stepdad needed more liquor, he'd call us to bring a truckload downtown."

"You knew how to drive?"

"We figured it out. Rita drove, and I shifted the gears. It took two of us, but we thought we were pretty tough."

My dad always said I needed to toughen up. Maybe I could bootleg whiskey.

Instead, my sister and brothers came home and headed straight to their rooms. I took a handful of cheese and watched *Bewitched* reruns on TV. I liked the show, but I never could figure out how a sensitive witch ended up married to such a boring and colorless man.

Chapter 16

Toughness

I sneak out of the hotel room early. I'll wake Cole if I bang around in the kitchenette, and I want him to sleep for a few more hours. I leave a note telling him I'll be back soon and gently lift a bag of grapes from the fridge on my way out.

I drive toward the botanical gardens, but first, I fill my car at a gas station and get an iced tea.

In less than fifteen minutes, I turn into the botanical gardens parking lot. Pink from the sunrise saturates the air. The gardens haven't opened yet, but even the parking lot is beautiful. The nearby trees look like weeping willows, but their bark is bright green like they grew up in a swamp but retained the lichen after the water receded.

I end up sitting in my car a lot lately, temporarily unable to move. I arrive at any given destination, but I need to wait for my internal gears to shift before getting out of the car. Navigating the world sober takes a lot of energy. I need Cave Woman.

—⚉—

Dear Cave Woman,

I'm anxious, and it's too early to call anyone. I guess you're stuck with me.

You can always talk with me, even early in the morning.

That's funny. My mom used to say, "You can always call me. Just not early in the morning."

After a few hours' sleep, I woke up wondering how I got so screwed up when my mom was so encouraging and smart. I know my dad humiliated me often, but why didn't her love and protection outweigh my dad's belittling?

You were lucky to have each other. You're still lucky. You have ready access to all her best qualities, including her insight, compassion, and humor. Your mom gave you an inside track to some of the more beautiful aspects of humanity. Your dad played hot potato with his emotions and carried on the family tradition of passing trauma through the family line. He couldn't control you and your mom, and patriarchy taught him to break the resistance from anyone who dared think for themselves, especially women.

I think my father did break me. With people outside our family, he was friendly and exuberant. People always told me how charming he was, which only made me look like the villain when I was defensive or defiant. Mostly, he was combative with me, like I was his sparring partner. I heard phrases like these almost every day:

What are you smiling about?

Who do you think you are?

What's the big idea?

Don't look so shocked. I'm just kidding.

I'm only trying to help.

Don't be ridiculous.

Lazybones.

I'll give you something to cry about.

He'd bend the truth to cast me in an unflattering light in ways that were confounding and hard to dispute.

Sometimes he would look at me as if to say, "I'm going to get you," like a bully on a playground.

Do you hear similar refrains from the Unreliable Narrator?

I don't think so, but maybe. I guess, yes, I suppose I do. Oh, no. The icky words are coming from inside my brain. That makes me so angry and bitter, I wanna scream. Dread seems to tackle me at arbitrary times of the day and night. Like a sudden downburst of horridness hits out of nowhere and flattens me. I feel short of breath and defeated.

Is this how I feel when the Unreliable Narrator has struck?

What do you think?

I think I need to fire the Unreliable Narrator right now.

Noticing the dialogue coming from the Unreliable Narrator speeds things along.

What can I do right now?

To ease the dread, go directly to the one in trouble. Make the decision to tell the terrified, helpless, younger versions of you, they're out of danger and safe. And then send them off to have the most exuberant and playful day imaginable.

Are you serious? That whole inner child thing seems kind of silly.

If the phrase "inner child" bothers you, call them your wee bairns or wild children. Or think of your inner children as energy that got cocooned at a younger age. Either way, you free the energy.

Maybe the inner child analogy is better than trying to picture energy. I like wild child. I'll give it a chance. I don't suppose it can hurt. But are they safe with me? I don't have much of a track record.

You're every age you've ever been, all at once. Healing entails soothing the younger parts of yourself and then sending them off to play. They're restless, bored, and angry. They were often helpless, and some are filled with rage. Free them from adult social restrictions and let them express their wild selves.

You want me to banish my inner children?

Hardly. They need to play, laugh, draw, captain pirate ships, and make mud pies. All the things children long for. You can create entire worlds where they can explore and have adventures. They can also cry or rage or break things. They get to do what you couldn't.

Being stuck inside an adult is constricting. They will ceaselessly fight to be at play in the wilds of your imagination and beyond.

I can see how being stuck inside of me is keeping them enraged. I can feel it. Can I really set them free?

Whenever you feel overwhelmed, you can be sure there's a wild child who needs to run free. While they're off playing, you get to recycle the genuine reactions they were denied during difficult times.

Oh, joy.

They're worth the effort. Plus, they'll be in charge until you set them free. They're a team and much stronger than you. But imagine how they'll feel after a day well played.

Imagine how you'll feel tonight with a passel of sleepy but contented wild ones.

How is this different from emotional flashbacks?

Run an experiment. Set them off to play and notice how you feel.

I don't have time to play. I'm not even sure I'd enjoy children's games.

Please remember, you're not going with them. Ask them what they'd like to do. Create the scene and encourage them to escape into play and exploration. They'll be safe, and you'll be free from their restlessness.

All this restlessness is from my wild children?

They're attempting to save you and themselves from being trapped in a confusing and tedious world overrun by restrictive rules.

Okay, okay, I'll give it a go.

I asked them where they want to spend the day and in my mind's eye, I see a big wooden ship. Cats and dogs lounge and play on the deck. I see kids climbing a rope to get on board before I even give them the go-ahead. I leave them with a protective crew. I feel foolish but miraculously less agitated. My stomach is calmer, and my chest feels more open.

I feel taller. A lot of trapped kid energy now roams free.

Dear Cave Woman,

Am I acting like an adult?

Being an adult is a lot easier without a passel of kids screaming to get out.

You're not kidding. I want to adult some more. I think I'll hit a meeting.

I look over my list of meetings and find one nearby that starts in thirty minutes. Pulling out of the parking lot without going into the botanical gardens feels a bit strange, but I know it's the best decision.

I need to learn a few adult things before the kids get home.

When the feeling of panic rises during the meeting, I reassure another wild child that we're okay and gently send them off to join the angelic crew on board the wooden ship. I feel calmer than I ever remember. Not all blissed out by any means, but calmer.

On the way back to the hotel, I pick up some half and half for Cole's coffee. We decided last night to visit a desert park outside the city. I'm excited and wait impatiently for him to finish an entire pot of coffee. His family has naturally low blood pressure and needs a gallon of coffee to get moving. When his mother couldn't sleep, she'd make a cup of coffee to cure her insomnia.

I leave the room, get two paper coffee cups and plastic lids from the lobby, return to the room, wordlessly fill them with what remains in the pot, hand them to Cole, and offer to drive.

Cole snorts, "Can't a man even finish his coffee around here?"

"Hey, I let you sleep in. I've been to a meeting already." I glare at him and shock myself by not backing down. "I think you can handle drinking your sacred coffee while I drive."

Cole picks up the to-go cups and with an attitude says, "Whatever."

We're having a spat, and we're still alive. We can argue without the fear of injuring each other, which is a relief and a tad invigorating.

I drive out of the city, and we gradually rise to a higher elevation. When the mountain plateaus, we stop at a ranger station to pay for a day pass. Inside are a few exhibits about the area.

While Cole pays for our passes, I'm drawn to a ranger with a swarm of red curly hair giving a demo with a live snake. As she handles the snake and brings it closer to the audience, I swoon and scream right along with the handful of children next to me. I get chills. I can't help it. The snake is both thrilling and sinister. The ranger says her name is Belinda, which means snake, but the kids and I are skeptical. We redeem our toughness with eye-rolling.

On our way back to the car, Cole and I are taken in by the view of the city, the valley below, and the tiny mountains on the other side of the Earth. It's seventy-three degrees with tall volcano-like clouds assembling in the west, which might indicate an afternoon thunderstorm and the makings of an ideal weather day.

As Cole drives, I look at the map of various hiking trails and find one that's three-quarters of a mile long. A perfect distance for an out-of-shape newly sober indoor type. I drink some water to hydrate.

We park and have the trail to ourselves. I tuck my water bottle in my backpack.

The whole outdoors smells like baking candy. Birds fly from cacti to cacti, checking us out and following along. Maybe they're looking for treats. It's hard to imagine they lack food with the high desert in bloom. The landscape looks like a tornado hit a fabric store and scattered the shreds on every stem, cacti, and bush. I feel like I can reach out and smear the colors like finger paints. It's a good thing the path is flat and well-maintained because I can't watch where I'm stepping; the riot of desert flowers takes my full attention.

I stop to take in the avant-garde scene and foolishly point and say, "Look at that!" over and over. I also stop and point to slyly catch my breath. Three-quarters of a mile is longer than I imagined. The water in my bottle is getting low, and I feel a slip of panic.

I turn my attention back to the flowering desert but sneak a look toward the parking lot. I can't believe there aren't thousands of people here to see this. Maybe the crowds are right behind us. I can see the entire trail and it looks like we're halfway done. Too late to turn back since the distance coming or going looks about the same. And then it hits me. The trail map didn't say three-quarters of a mile; it said 3.4 miles. On no, I can't do this. Can we call for help? Maybe for a helicopter or at least a golf cart. I explain my mistake to Cole, and he confirms that we can turn around, but the distance would be the same. He also laughs at my miscalculation. I hand him my backpack as payback, but I laugh too.

I'm not sure I can walk that far. Then I remember all the meetings where people said to pray. I think for a minute and say my very first prayer. I don't ask for transportation back to the car or for my water to miraculously multiply. I make it much simpler. I pray to keep from complaining. Help me, Great Whatever, help me not to moan, cry, or complain. Help me not utter a single grievance. I stand straighter and start walking.

I've put Cole through enough by promising to quit drinking so many times. I don't want to dampen the joy of witnessing a blooming desert on an ideal winter day.

When I feel distress, I imagine a restless wild child running free. I reassure her we're fine and she can always find me. I give her the go-ahead to go off-trail. She picks monkeyflowers and bluebells, kisses burrowing owls on the head, and swoops and nosedives with the hawks. She makes scientific observations and takes notes. The view is spectacular, and I'll get her back to the car where I have a jug filled with ice water.

I struggle to keep up with Cole. Just as my panic eases, my water runs out, and I scream silently a few times and ask my crowd of kids to scream too. We make a game of it.

We make it back to the car with a lot of silent celebrating. My plucky children and I are proud of ourselves, but we don't brag. We talk it over and decide bragging would just be complaining after the fact. They're tired, so I send them back to the wooden ship for a snack and a nap. Once I'm done imagining, I'm not tired at all.

Cole wants to hike another trail. I beg off and sit in the car and write to Cave Woman.

—⁓—

Dear Cave Woman,

Is this all I need to feel good? Free my wild children to have adventures? Reassure them they're safe and loved, and then I'll feel better?

Remember, difficult situations got tucked safely away when they were too intense to fully feel in the moment. When the child who felt that pain is free, safe, and exploring, you're free to work on recovery. You can feel anything now that you're a sober adult.

I was such a lousy guardian for the younger parts of me. This might take some practice.

Even an imperfect present, with an imperfect but imaginative adult, is far better than being stuck in a child's intense reaction.

And please notice when you feel good. If you don't take note when you feel content, you'll have nothing to build on. As they rediscover the world, so will you.

—⁓—

The clouds get darker and closer. The moment I wonder if Cole will be safe walking during a thunderstorm, he returns. He knows the wilderness much better than I do.

He leans over and kisses me, and we both smile shyly.

He drives slowly, and we eat at a Hawaiian restaurant. I ask the woman behind the counter why the desert in bloom wasn't a huge draw, and she says, "This is nothing. Wait until the rainy season. Then you'll really see something."

"I'm from a very snowy area, and I guess seeing flowers during the winter is miraculous," I say and smile.

I love this day.

Witches

It's late, the bar is closed, and I'm sitting in a lounge chair by the pool, hugging my backpack. I've heard of restless legs syndrome, but I think I have restless body syndrome. Sleep experts online recommend getting out of bed if you can't sleep, so I did. I put on the thin grey sweatshirt and sweatpants I'd left on a chair the night before. I stole a pair of Cole's socks in case it was cool outside. The dim outdoor lights point toward the ground and glow like candlelight. Unseen frogs and crickets conduct the background music. Maybe they like to stay hidden, too.

I feel calmer being near water, even by a swimming pool.

I open my backpack and open my notebook to a fresh page.

———〰———

Dear Cave Woman,

I feel like half of me is okay, and half of me is monstrously inept. **Only half? We're making progress.**

Trying to hide my imperfection only makes me more obviously imperfect. I just want to hide all the damn time, even sober. Why did I feel so unsafe in the boring old suburbs as a kid? Why did I feel so powerless to change anything?

All children need safety and security. Your mom gave you all the safety and security she could, but she had very little power. Few women did when you were little.

When did women have power?

For most of history, women had equal power. Power wasn't divided by gender. All people in my community were equal. We wouldn't have survived any other way.

Were women the healers?

In my community, anyone could be a healer. Later in history, the healing arts become the purview of women. But that was stolen, too.

How? What's an example?

For example, millions of healers, mostly women, were murdered by profiteers for freely practicing the healing arts. It started in Europe, but the killing spread throughout the world, like greed.

Why?

Profit, religious persecution, and control.

We lost our healing knowledge for money. That makes me livid. How did they get away with murdering so many?

They called healers witches and taught people to be afraid of anyone who practiced natural medicine. The capitalist class, or what you call patriarchy, feared the power in healing. Each time a life was taken, valuable healing knowledge moved further underground.

No wonder we're depressed, addicted, and in pain. We've lost our knowledge and capacity to care for ourselves. Patriarchy won by killing the healers and terrorizing everyone else into submission.

Not entirely. People can still learn to heal themselves and assist others. And every day you're sober, you regain a bit of power and elicit a faint memory of your natural abilities.

History is validating. The oppression continues, and the violence is far from over. Addiction makes sense in a historical context. I feel oddly relaxed when I should be horrified.

The truth resonates even when it's complicated. How does your body feel?

My stomach and jaw are relaxed. I feel solid yet clear. The information resonates, but my mind is distrustful.

Your Unreliable Narrator was scripted to reject your own healing sensitivities, installed by those who want to maintain control, keeping you submissive and powerless. The self-defeating and self-sabotaging narration keeps you in that state.

Wouldn't self-sabotage be unnatural?

Of course. Self-loathing is unnatural, and everything about you will holler to regain self-regard. The script of the Unreliable Narrator denies your own gut sense and pushes you toward capitulating to authority.

And my mighty weapon is sensitivity? Is patriarchy where perfectionism and self-pressure come from?

Yes, to both of your questions. In my time, sensitivity was a highly prized trait. But sensitivity is not the right word. People like you were valued for their keen perception. High Perceivers kept the reckless majority of us safe.

A High Perceiver can read a situation in a second, know what's out of place, know who's mad at whom, and glean any threats.

High Perceivers noticed when one of our own had slipped into self-loathing or become disconnected from our community.

High Perceivers were our first line of defense against liars and manipulators.

But it's tiring to be a High Perceiver.

Exactly, I knew you'd recognize yourself. High Perceivers processed a lot of information and were protected and trained to handle their gift early.

How did you protect them? Can you give me an example?

For example, when we traveled in groups, we'd rotate the High Perceivers from the outside of the group back to the middle so half the High Perceivers could take breaks. We had to encourage them to take breaks as often as possible. Most of us goofed off a lot and were a hardier bunch, but truly we weren't safe without them.

Being a High Perceiver takes a toll, especially when you're bullied and abused for your keen awareness, the exact skill that makes you valuable to a community.

Because your High Perceiver skills were not appreciated or cultivated, you often don't realize what you've picked up on until days or weeks later. We'll change that so you can process what you perceive more readily.

What else does being a High Perceiver get me?

Intuitive hits about the future and an ability to talk with the plants, the fungi, the water, the animals, the cosmos, and laugh about the curiosity of it all.

Will I dance naked with the goddesses of yesteryear and sing with the fairies and angels?

You joke, but before patriarchy, we revered the feminine in all things. Women are the source of life and were once respected and venerated. With the ability to give life came the ability to expand life. When women lost their power, all humanity suffered.

With the loss of genuine power, all that remains is the illusion of control.

So, we're all powerless except for a few control freaks?

Not at all. Control can never replace true power. Most of your people have hidden their power so deep inside, they've forgotten it's there. People gain control over others in small and large arenas and—

—ɯ—

I stop writing for a minute as people pass by. They arrive back tipsy after a night out, some laughing, some arguing. It's interesting how people react differently to alcohol. I was a happy, chatty drunk before I became a stay-at-home drinker; after humiliating myself one too many times.

—ɯ—

Dear Cave Woman,

Pardon the interruption.

In modern times, do only the strongest and cruelest survive?

No, that's a myth. Survival doesn't require being strong and cruel. Survival requires the ability to adapt and cooperate. Competition among humans is deadly because ultimately, humans rely on each other for survival.

But humans throw each other under the bus all the time, and we just keep making more people.

Yes, but not working together will eventually lead to the end of the human species on Earth.

I hate this so much. I hate humanity for killing itself when we could do so much if we worked together and didn't let a few rich people make all the rules. I don't want to witness our destruction. I might as well start drinking again.

Which would be doing what?

Ah, crap…killing myself and not working with others to find solutions.

You got it. Your worldview is skewed. See if you can find a different perspective once you've been in recovery a bit longer.

How do people break each other down?

People manipulate through lies, threats, gossip, and propaganda. Even apologies can be a form of manipulation. People can manipulate entire regions of the world and gain control to kill and torture millions.

Control is having my wellbeing taken away and having it offered back for a price?

How awful. What is *real* power like?

Real power transforms trauma into innovation. Real power is creative in a way that doesn't intentionally traumatize or exploit anyone. Real power unites and encourages wholeness through play, rest, work, and community.

A rising tide lifts all boats?

Exactly. True power comes when you invite the disparate parts of yourself to work together and reveal wholeness. Wholeness creates lasting success.

How do I get me some power?

Finding a bit of your true nature here and there and never relying on one specific person or one ideology is a healthy way to build your internal hive. Regaining true power is the most radical act on planet Earth.

Hey, that's one way I'm strong. I've never followed anyone blindly. It's cost me a lot, but I think it might be a strength. But I'm weird and awkward. I have outlandish dreams of how much better the world could be. I think that excludes me from most groups.

Formal groups, yes. But don't be afraid to dream outlandish dreams. Almost every innovation has been met with skepticism and derision. Being weird is what the world needs. Awkward is weird's second cousin. Relish them all.

You want me to love being weird and awkward?

The more you love and appreciate your unique inner hive,

the more resources you're able to reclaim. You'll find people that complement your wholeness. You'll find weird, awkward, outlandish, innovative dreamers. You'll find home.

The sky is getting lighter. I feel sleepy. Why do I often feel like I can finally sleep just as the night is over?

You've released the pressure to fall asleep simply because it was nighttime.

So, this is what depressurization feels like. I can see why you call it magic. This might take practice.

Chapter 17

Shaking Helps

Maggie and I meet at a French restaurant with small glass-topped tables and tiny uncomfortable iron café chairs. Her long, curly black hair solidly frames her grounded disposition. We'd become friends at a marketing conference here in Phoenix five years ago and kept in touch sporadically. The friendly lilt of her voice could get her a successful career as a hypnotist. I'll need lots of iced tea to keep from getting too relaxed. I'm still nervous talking with someone who isn't in recovery and who may not understand that I'm a bit insane right now.

"I have a new grandbaby, and we've moved our business to a much larger space," she started, with little prompting.

I love people who can take the conversation. My shoulders relax. "Oh, tell me all about it. Any pictures?"

First, she asks about me. I tell her about the new job in Haiti but leave out the part about my one month of sobriety. She has many stories and updates. I'm grateful to listen, relax, and enjoy. She tells me of tragedies and triumphs with admirable clarity about lessons learned and dreams for the future. I want to live in Phoenix forever and have lively lunches with generous friends.

"When can you and Cole come over?"

I hesitate to make plans. What if I feel shaky? What would I say if they offer me a drink? What if they offered me a drink and I couldn't say no? But I want to do something normal with kind people, so I surprise myself and say, "Friday evening?"

"We have family coming over that night. I'm not sure why, but they always seem to be at my house." She laughs, but her house has always been the hub of family gatherings.

"I know why," I say with a smile. She'd taken many hard knocks as her children grew and still managed to start a successful business and create closeness with her children and grandchildren that anyone on Earth would admire. "It's all you." I continue, "Cole and I found the best Italian deli since I lived in NYC. We could pick up a few subs or pizzas and come by for lunch on Sunday?"

"That could work," she says, nodding her head yes.

Ordinary lunches with friends used to sound so boring to me. Camaraderie always came from a bottle. Now I can enjoy myself without drinking and ending up with a hangover. I can feel intimacy and friendship, free for the taking.

After lunch, I put the key in the ignition, and my hands start shaking. Maybe a little too much iced tea. I step on the brake to put the car in reverse, and my leg shakes so hard it bounces off the brake pedal. I throw the car back in park. The shaking spreads from my legs and arms to my torso. I feel like I'm at the epicenter of an earthquake. Isn't it too late for the DTs? I think about taking a cab to a doctor, but the shaking lessens. Nothing like worry about a doctor's bill to shut down symptoms. I write Cave Woman instead.

—⚊—

Dear Cave Woman,

Why did I shake so bad after a lovely lunch with a lovely friend?

Visiting a doctor is still a good idea, but the shaking wasn't about withdrawal.

Your body was poised for danger and is now releasing the energy of a potential survival response. Shaking allowed your body to release the pent-up adrenaline.

Part of me felt threatened?

Your Survival Brain is always on the lookout for possible threats. New experiences are scanned for potential threats. Without alcohol—or the promise of alcohol—all new experiences will be treated as suspect. Allowing the shaking helped reset your nervous system.

I feel like a feral child learning the rules of polite society for the first time.

You sat there pleased as punch, having a nice lunch with lots of eye contact, while a feral wildness inside you felt trapped like a baby monkey surrounded by wolverines. Now that the "danger" has passed, your body shakes, just like an animal's body shakes post-danger.

I'll be shaking all the time.

The longer you remain sober, the more easily you'll assimilate novel experiences. Let yourself shake, exaggerate it if you can. Go with it and appreciate your feral self for all its uncivilized, rule-breaking originality. Reassure your wild children that a little socializing is fine. Let them know you'll never burden them with the expectation of being a social butterfly. Let them go wild whenever possible.

Chapter 18

Potent Fuel

Cole finally spoke with one of the people sponsoring our trip to Haiti. The man said the information we need is contained in a letter sent to our hotel. When Cole hangs up, a dark look crosses his face. Neither one of us says anything out loud. Instead of discussing whether we should be skeptical about hearing the equivalent of, "The check is in the mail," we walk to a nearby park to play Frisbee golf.

When we get to the park, I learn quickly that I hate Frisbee golf. It's difficult and tedious, and I don't have the patience right now. In a fit of tantrum, I offer the Frisbees to a group of teenagers passing by.

Cole looks shocked, and I'm too mad to care.

"Do you want to play with us?" one of them asks Cole. I think they feel sorry for Cole and my temper tantrum.

"Sure, why not?" Cole replies, happy to avoid me for a bit.

I walk over to a large willow tree, sit, and watch them play for a while. They're laughing so hard one ends up rolling on the ground in hysterics. I hated the game, but I admit they're fun to watch. They lighten my mood.

I have a notebook and pen in my backpack.

—◊—

Dear Cave Woman,

This might be a crazy question, but is it possible to have fun getting sober?

It's not a crazy question at all. Fun is a key ingredient for success. Modern humans often overlook the value of fun. I know you're worried about the future, but also notice your fascination with the whys and hows of addiction. Curiosity is one of the most potent fuels on Earth.

I never would have associated the words fun or fascinated with getting sober. But I admit it. I'm interested in finding out if I can pull this off. I'm curious how anyone gets through life without alcohol. You've made me interested in recovery. I never could have done this without you.

Well, thank you but—

But I'd like to talk about money. Money baffles me. I've had so many ideas. I've made a lot of money for other people, but my own ideas yielded very little success.

You worked your ideas from your head only, which left you disconnected from your Creative Genius and ignoring the clues from your resourceful body. You inevitably ran out of steam.

I wasn't having fun, was I?

No, you felt pressure, not fun. A good idea is like a car with no fuel. You can push on the bumper and get a bit of movement, but it's a waste of energy. For success that doesn't

require a lifetime of grueling work, it needs an element of felicity.

I've taken everything too seriously?

Precisely. You either need to bring levity to your work or balance it out with fun on the side.

I believe that, but I feel bad if I'm enjoying work. So many people hate work.

Welcome to your world. But feeling bad about enjoying work while others suffer misses the point. The world would be a vastly different place if work revolved around collaboration.

And feeling bad?

An old habit.

Gawd, another one?

You were programmed to feel bad for feeling good. Free yourself from the idea that feeling good has an upper limit. Work or service can't always equal drudgery, including changing the world for the better.

You now have first-hand experience navigating a significant change. You found curiosity and some enjoyment along the way. These ingredients work like magic on reconfiguring old habits.

—⚍—

Cole lays down on the ground next to me, sweaty but smiling. I scoot closer to him, and he turns on his side with his head propped in one hand. We look at each other, and I know he is going to tell me something I don't want to hear.

"No, don't tell me," I beg.

"I have to, Sil." He rolls over on his back and looks at the gathering clouds. "I talked to Spence this morning, and my old job is available. The guy who took it skipped town. So I'm going back."

"Can't we stay here?" We both know our trip to Haiti is not happening, and we don't even mention it.

"I don't think I could take the heat in the summers. And what would I do?"

"You could be a supportive partner. You could get work here. Maybe even something you like." I'm furious again.

"I followed you here, didn't I?" Cole says in an unusually biting tone. He's mad, too.

"My whole life has become an apology for getting us into this mess. Why would you say that to me?"

"Someone has to be responsible."

"That's low. Your responsibility is so noble it's exhausting. Doesn't how I feel matter?"

"Our money is almost gone. I'm going back. I'll stay with Spence until I can rent us a place. That is if you want to come back at all."

"Are you trying to make me mad? Do you want me to stay here permanently?"

"That's up to you, but I'm leaving."

He's made up his mind, and I vexingly can't convey how much I want to live here. I seethe, feeling like a clamp is tightening at the back of my neck. "I can't go back. I have to stay. Otherwise, I'll drink again. I like it here. I like us better here."

"Don't get upset, Sil. I've thought of that. I found a short-term rental for you. It's nice. You can stay here for three more months, go to your meetings, and I'll find us a place to live. Then you can come home."

"I still don't believe work is the real reason you're leaving. You could find work here.

Why won't you tell me the real reason?" I plead.

"Think about it, okay?" He doesn't answer my question. I want to scream. But what I think about is the nearest liquor store. Bright and shiny and waving me home. I know I need to stay here to get more recovery time, but why can't we both stay?

I stuff my notebook and water bottle in my backpack and stomp back toward the hotel. For the first time since we met, I don't care if he follows me or not.

I think about ways I can convince him to stay. Once he's back at his job, he'll never leave. I hear him come back while I'm attempting to cool off in the shower. I don't have to ask what emotion I'm feeling. I'm so mad I could stamp my foot and rip a hole in the bottom of the tub. Breathe. Feel the anger. Let it disperse. Nope. That didn't work. I'll just stay mad. Maybe I even need to yell.

Instead, we do what we've always done and get through the evening: we don't talk, we don't yell, we don't get anywhere.

When we get in bed, I say through a clenched jaw, "This is so unfair. I don't like how we got here but I love it here. I have friends. I'm in recovery. Doesn't that mean anything to you?"

"It means a lot to me. But I have to do my job. I'm freaked out about money and this is right in front of me."

"No, I'm right in front of you and I need you here."

"There's nothing for me here."

"Does that include me?"

"I didn't mean it that way. Look, I can only take one trauma at a time. Give me a chance to start over."

"You mean maybe we could come back?"

"I don't know, Sil. I have to go and that's all I know."

"You are so mean."

"If that's how you feel, I'll leave right now." He sits up in bed and starts putting his clothes back on.

I sit up and whisper yell, "This is why we don't argue or talk or figure things out together. This is why things get so messed up. We don't talk about anything serious. You won't fight. You bail on every argument. It's not fair to threaten to leave. We have to learn to fight."

"Okay, we'll learn to fight."

"You mean it?"

"I promise we can fight more. How's that?" Cole says sarcastically and rolls his eyes.

"A cop out."

"I know. I hate to fight. I'm no good at it," he concedes.

"I hear the make-up sex is pretty good," I offer.

"I'm still mad."

"I'm still mad, too."

"What now?"

"We stay mad and see what happens. I guess. I don't know." Cole lays back in the bed. "I'm falling asleep. Can we fight more tomorrow?" Cole pleads.

I smile but don't let him hear it in my voice. "I guess that'll have to do for now. Good night, Mr. Boring Responsibility."

"Good night, Ms. Starry-eyed Dreamer."

I turn away. I'm shaking because I think we just survived our first major fight. Maybe there's hope we can talk things through.

Basket of Rocks

Cole is asleep in minutes and I feel resentful at his ability to fall asleep so soon after fighting. I want to kick my legs against the mattress until he wakes up, let him fall asleep, then kick the mattress again. I hate lying here, so I huff loudly and go to the bathroom. I dry out the tub and line it with pillows to write to Cave Woman.

—⟶⟵—

Dear Cave Woman,

Cole wants to return to the frozen north. I never want to go back.

We've given up on the job overseas. It breaks my heart for Maddy and Cole. The despair feels urgent.

Let despair take the pen.

—⟶⟵—

As I write out my despair, it feels like I've dumped out a basket of trapped and restless snakes. fear takes the pen, then rage, and then I tap a vein of sadness and the tears begin. I get out of the tub to blow my nose and I scrape my back on the faucet, and it feels like I've been stabbed in the back. The pain is intense and infuriating and I instantly want to drink. I slither onto the floor and writhe until the pain eases. I want to crush the faucet with my feet but instead grab a towel and wail on the defenseless bathmat. When I'm done, I sit cross-legged and prop up the notebook against my knee.

—⟶⟵—

Dear Cave Woman,

Despair had a lot to say. So did fear, rage, and sadness. Busy night, but I feel less anxious and less sad. But I can't do this every night.

And you won't need to. Pens, pencils, and paper are comforting to you, giving just enough support to write openly. Before you explore any emotion, make sure to evoke a comforting memory, comforting daydream, or hold an object that helps you feel supported.

If I already feel comforted, why would I have to explore the emotions?

To help garner insight. Emotions only trip you up if you ignore them. Did writing it out help?

It did, and the craving is gone. I can't believe I planned on going out in the morning with a basket full of raging snakes.

What do you think might have happened?

I'm not sure. Maybe I would have yelled at another driver, maybe some road rage, maybe a car accident, maybe a trip to the liquor store.

I'm proud of you for taking the time to feel and for writing it out.

Ah, shucks.

Walking around without a sense of your current thoughts and emotions can feel like a basket full of rocks dangling from your waist. Let's leave the snakes out of it. Snakes are wonderful creatures and get enough bad press.

A basket full of rocks would make it hard to move.

Yes, it'd be hard to move without getting irritated and exhausted. Your fellow alcoholics often think they make a conscious choice to end up at the liquor store. But more than likely, they left home with the emotional equivalent of a basket filled with rocks.

I won't drink but I still feel churned up.

That's natural. You're settling a bit at a time. Rivers turn muddy during the spring runoff, but the water always clears.

The mud doesn't bother the rivers. A bit of settled mud, rich with nutrients, provides a toehold for plants to grow. The vegetation, in turn, keeps the banks in place, allowing the fish and wildlife to thrive.

I get so bogged down.

Rivers just keep flowing, confident that clarity is right around the bend. Emotions sift through you and sometimes leave helpful information. Not permitting them to sift, bogs you down.

I'd like to run clear and go with the flow and all that. Anything is better than willpower, which hasn't done much for me.

Willpower only lasts when you're focused on control, which is not only exhausting, it's impossible. The minute you drop your focus, you slip. Your emotions want to walk beside you, not trip you up. You've had enough of that in your drinking days.

Very funny. I didn't know you had a sense of humor, too. What if an emotion wants attention and I'm at work or at a restaurant?

If you don't have time to write, acknowledge the emotions. Send a bit of appreciation for their protective nature and their willingness to be on call, like your very own set of superheroes.

I get up off the floor and grab a hand towel as I leave the bathroom. I roll some ice in a towel. Lying next to Cole, I wiggle onto the towel where my back met the faucet. At first it hurts worse but as I relax, the pain eases.

Recycling Bin

I wake up a few hours later to a wet spot in the bed. I wonder if Cole peed the bed. Or maybe I peed the bed. I'm confused for a moment then remember the towel with ice for my back. I laugh thinking about telling Cole I thought he peed the bed. We could have another fight. I better let him sleep. Where did I leave my notebook? That's right, in the bathroom. I remember Cole is leaving. I'm awake and annoyed. I might as well sit on the bathroom floor again.

—⁓—

Dear Cave Woman,

I've decided one part of the Survival Brain functions like a recycling bin in need of a regular clean-out.

That's a good analogy. Your Survival Brain safely cocoons emotions too complex to feel during a difficult experience. These emotionally charged memories affect your body and mind.

And contribute to physical pain and addictions?

Correct.

What about emotional flashbacks?

Emotional flashbacks indicate that you're ready to process an emotion.

But taking out the recycling can be painful.

Less so when you understand what is happening.

Just the other day, I remembered a time when my dad humiliated my brother for getting a C on his report card. My dad got all Cs, but apparently that's another story. The memory of my humiliated brother sitting on the couch was painful to recall. I felt hot rocks of shame in my chest, and I found myself craving Hostess Ho Hos. You know, the kind you can unroll? I wanted a whole box of Hostess Ho Hos. I don't even like Hostess Ho Hos. They're kind of waxy tasting.

Hostess Ho Hos are what you ate as you listened to your father berate your brother, which set a pattern to eat sugar when you felt or witnessed humiliation. That old memory came up for recycling and the habit to suppress caused the craving for Hostess Ho Hos. You're not letting the emotion-laden memory get recycled. You fought against feeling the memory.

I didn't know I was so opposed to recycling.

You're not. It's just a habit you learned, a habit you share with most of the modern world. A habit can change.

How do I take out the recycling?

Let's start by putting all your thoughts, concerns, and worries in a soundproof booth.

Done. What's next?

What would your guess be?

If I'm following correctly, I experience difficulties and traumas system-wide. So, healing would need to be system-wide or felt as a full-body experience.

Good point. I keep forgetting you're still learning to feel present in your body.

Okay. Can you tap your feet and hands to start feeling into your body?

I can't. I hate this.

Remember your evening at the botanical gardens and the flamenco guitar?

I do.

How does that memory feel?

Soft and bright. Kind of silky. Okay, I think that helped. I'm here.

Excellent. And what could you ask yourself next?

If I'm mad, sad, glad, or afraid and feeling the emotion as a physical sensation.

And if you can't name the emotion?

I'm not sure.

You could just let it be energy without a name.

Oh, okay. That works for me. Right now, I'm smad; part mad, part sad. Now I feel the emotion and see if it moves or shifts?

Yes, and instead of tensing against an emotion, you're going to breathe toward where you feel the sensation.

Won't that expand it?

It might, but breathing into the emotional sensation will ultimately open a space for insight to flow in and help all emotions flow more readily.

And if I dare to breathe toward this smad in my body, then what?

What would you like to do?

Umm, I could do what your people did and sing, shout, dance, cry, or whatever else the emotional energy wants to do?

Would you like me to look away?

Yes, please. Give me a minute.

Take all the time you need.

Dear Cave Woman,

I'm back. I felt the sadness in my stomach and breathed into it like a balloon. It dissipated quickly. I felt mad in my legs. Breathing into my legs kind of required expanding my entire body like a big tent. I wanted to stop because I felt even angrier, but I kept breathing into it as it moved to my hips and into my chest. Then I wanted to help the anger act itself out.

And?

I acted out chopping off my dad's head for humiliating my brother. Then I imagined people all over the world dancing around baskets filled with the chopped off heads of sankes. I shook my fists and laughed with cartoonish glee. Now, I feel softer, less tense. Took less than a minute.

But am I creating more violence in the world by imagining such violent things?

You're reducing violence by acting out your emotions and not taking them out on others or on the natural world.

Did you gain any insights?

Feeling is freeing and lessens tension.

Feeling is freeing. Feeling an emotion is not complicated. That idea might take some getting used to. Modern people can complicate a blueberry.

But if it's freeing to feel, why does it often feel like my emotions are trying to torture me?

Because you never learned how to digest experiences. You never learned that your emotions can illuminate a situation.

I'm embarrassed to say I'm still afraid of my feelings.

It's what you've been taught. You're not alone. Many people lack the ability to understand these dedicated and lion-hearted protectors. No matter how deeply you've buried your feelings, they'll never give up on you. Their loyalty is unwavering.

Can I drink emotions away?

No, my devious fox. You gave that strategy your best and it still didn't work. You can pour addictive substances over unresolved feelings or attempt to ignore them with obsessive behaviors, but the recycling will continue to pile up.

I remember you saying we either stuff emotions or push them off on someone else. I called it playing a game of emotional hot potato. I get it, but can you give me some examples?

Parents who don't understand their own anger use it like a weapon and raise angry children, or children who are easily defeated by anger, or both.

Teachers who don't understand their own fear, bully fearful students.

Friends who don't understand how to handle envy can become cruel, arrogant, or unavailable.

Being emotionally illiterate is like being a cat with monstrously sharp claws and no idea how to retract them. The cuts and deep wounds devastate all within scratching distance. Including themselves.

For all this effort at controlling our feelings, we sure seem bad at it.

Just terrible, I agree. Your world is a virtual blood bath caused by misunderstood emotions. In some cases, this leads to a literal blood bath. If your people put one-tenth of the effort toward understanding emotions as they do toward fighting emotions, the world would transform phenomenally.

What happens to all my unresolved emotions?

You turn some of that toxicity on yourself, which can turn into dangerously high blood pressure or an inability to get out of bed for ten days. Or you can't think coherently and act out.

Okay, so all this time I thought I was very in touch with my emotions, was I really in touch with fighting against them?

Often that was the case, yes. Very good.

What do I do with all those thoughts, concerns, and worries in the soundproof booth?

What would you like to do?

Good question. Let me ponder that a bit. I get to choose?

You get to choose.

I'll leave them there for now. I feel good. My body feels like it's thrumming.

Oh, I like the word thrumming, that's your emotions guidance system going back online.

Your Survival Brain likes when you bring all your resources on board.

—⟋⟍—

Sober Sex

When Cole wakes up, we make up and have our first go at sober sex. First, we brush our teeth. I've never believed movies where the lovers wake up and start kissing. Morning breath is awful.

Things progress okay until I start laughing. I don't know why I'm laughing but I can't stop. The idea of sex without wine seems absurd.

"Will we get the hang of make-up sex the more we fight?" Cole asks and we laugh, get out of bed, and dress for breakfast.

Over coffee for Cole and tea and oatmeal for me, I ask Cole if he'll go look at the short-term rental unit and see how it looks in person. I don't want to think about him leaving, but I also don't want to go back to the frozen north.

When he's at the rental office, he calls and says it looks nice and I can move in in three days. He's starting the paperwork and will be home later.

I reluctantly agree. I'm relieved to be staying but wish more than anything Cole would stay, too.

"You'll like it. The buildings seem new and it's next to a large park. Okay?"

"I said okay. Go ahead," I bark. But I want to say, why can't we make a life here where I finally got sober and where I have sober friends? I appreciate all he's done and all he is doing for me. For us.

I can't get him to stay. I feel like a failure. I fall on the bed. I'm ugly, I'm stupid, I'm a fool. My Unreliable Narrator has a field day.

Trading Addictions

Packing doesn't take long. We check out of the hotel and hit two different dollar stores for kitchen and bathroom items. I get a pack of bright orange bath towels, dish soap, a few utensils, two knives—one small, one large—two plates, two mugs, four glasses, and a pan. I forgot cleaning supplies, so we stop at another dollar store. This place is crawling with dollar stores. I also get cleaning supplies, a broom, a dustpan, and laundry soap.

The short-term rental complex is less like a hotel and more suburban than I imagined. The lawn is manicured with a sidewalk that meanders like a stream. Cole and I debate if this would help or hinder coming home drunk.

The complex consists of six two-story buildings. I'm relieved my front door is near the pool. I also like that the sliding glass door in the back has a view of the park. I wonder if Cole picked the one near the pool because he knew I'd like it best. My heart softens a bit more.

The apartment is about the same size as our hotel room, but with a separate bedroom. The kitchenette, large enough for one person, has a small stove, a tiny stainless-steel sink, and a tall, light blue refrigerator. The light-brown plastic-covered couch looks brand new. Cole says no one is living above me, which I appreciate.

We go out for an early dinner. I want to eat all the time and I'm concerned I'll eat nonstop once Cole leaves. We walk through the park that evening to a grocery store and I buy fruits and vegetables to encourage a healthy diet. Once Cole is asleep, I give myself a few hours to fall asleep before I search out Cave Woman.

—⚏—

Dear Cave Woman,

I heard at a meeting that once you give up one addiction, another takes its place.

Is that true?

It does seem to happen quite a bit. Trading alcohol for sugar and cigarettes. Trading drugs for brief dalliances. Or cocaine for adrenaline-inducing behaviors, like gambling, thrill-seeking, dangerous sports, or manipulating and controlling other people.

I've known many people addicted to adrenaline. People who hike dozens of miles a day or fly precariously down mountain trails on bikes. I suppose an addiction to exercise is more socially acceptable, but I bet it's still painful. Far more people share addiction than anyone realizes. Can emotions be addictive also?

People can become habituated to an emotional state when they don't know how to work with the emotion. For example, if a person is continually angry at work but finds themselves feeling empty during weekends, they may unconsciously long for a hit of anger.

This happened to Cole. He took a rare day off and seemed out of sorts. His job made him angry a lot.

"Do you miss getting pissed off?" I asked.

He surprised us both by saying, "Yes, I want someone to call about something idiotic and make me furious. I feel empty."

Cole was habituated to a hit of anger. Without work, he'd look for excuses to fill that void. Emotions bind to the same cell-receptor sites as heroin. Feeling emotions is so vital to our survival that we're rewarded for paying attention. Unfortunately, the "emptiness" gets confused with a need for more anger. Just like with alcohol.

How can I prevent myself from getting a fix from an emotion?

People believe they obsess about a topic because the situation demands that much attention. Actually, they're replaying it for a hit of anger, fear, or whichever emotion the thoughts invoke. Look at the problem, not the guards who stepped up to help.

Let me tell you a story.

A man in my tribe once lost a knife. He stomped about looking for it and yelling threats if it wasn't found. We laughed at first, thinking it was a joke. When days passed and he still railed about the lost knife, we became concerned.

He would not come to the fire in the evenings or share his dreams in the morning. This scared us because we knew how to keep our psyches from getting clogged up and he refused to let us assist him.

Whenever he thought about the knife, he became angry.

Whenever he became emotional, he thought about anger, which led to thoughts about the missing knife.

No matter what he thought about or felt, he'd run into the chain that had linked the missing knife with anger.

Someone, I don't remember who, finally brought him to the fire. We danced and sang. We cried. He cried. Not for the missing knife. We could always make another one. Even he knew that. He cried with relief when he glimpsed the mind-looping as nothing more than an obsession we could help him ease. We all cried for how easily our minds can get stuck on a single topic and distort our perception. When thoughts and emotions become entwined, they can seem as strong as a chain. And almost as unbreakable.

Chapter 19

Live Wire

Since Cole is returning north, he'll need another car. We sold his old car right before we left. He knows what make and model he wants, and we end up stuck at the dealership for five hours. We wait impatiently in a large room with three brightly polished cars and a glossy floor. I smell strawberry air freshener, but I can't find the source. I feel like we're posing for a corporate brochure, unable to move until they get just the right shot. There's a mini fridge with cold water bottles and I drink four. At least going to the bathroom gives me something to do.

Our salesman sits in his glass-enclosed office, doing nothing.

"Do you think they're doing a background check?" I ask Cole.

"I'm sure. Or seeing if we'll break down and admit we're criminals."

"I can see why people would break. There's nothing to do here. It's like time has slowed down and the air freshener is laced with monotony. I'll admit I'm a criminal if we can get out of here."

We don't talk about Cole leaving or why I'm staying. I'm afraid I'll cry. I'm afraid I'll scream and beg.

"I have a confession," I say with rocks in my stomach.

"Okaaayyy," Cole says slowly.

"I think I learned in my family that the husband needs to be coddled. We were always pacifying my dad. But you're a good man and you can handle difficult discussions. We can learn to talk about how we really feel. I don't bite, right?"

"Do we really have to?" he says half-joking. "I hate talking about how I feel. I don't know how."

"How about you talk about your gut reactions and I'll talk about feelings?"

"My gut says that doesn't sound too terrible."

"I get the impression I could do or say whatever I wanted, and you'd stick with me as long as we didn't have to talk about things," I say.

"Would that be so bad?" He grins hopefully, but I have more I need to say.

"Maddy might think so. My liver might think so. Let's just talk things through. I promise we don't have to talk them to death." I take a deep breath and add, "The worst part of you leaving is not including me in the decision. I decided we should go on this wild goose chase and I take responsibility. But we need to decide things together. Okay?"

"Do you have a pamphlet I can read?" he jokes.

"I'll make one and give you a copy."

The salesman finally brings the keys and Cole drives his new car back to my new place. I follow. He packs and the next morning I walk him to his car at 6:00 in the morning. He sits in the driver's seat, raring to go. I stand by his open window and inhale the smell of his shave cream. I need to speak quickly before he takes off and apologize again for getting us into this mess.

"I'm sorry for everything. This whole mess. Is there any way I can make it up to you?"

He could get in a brutal parting shot and fear grips my stomach like a vice.

Cole says, "You already are. Just keep doing what you're doing."

Tears hover in my throat, but I'll save those for later. I feel like a responsible grown up, real and present. Not lost or grasping for answers.

I kiss him and want to drag him back to bed, but he's ready to drive. I was mad he was leaving, now I'm mad he's in such a hurry. I get mad a lot lately. As he drives away, I cry for a bit but honestly, I'm relieved. I'll miss him, but sometimes I feel like an angry live wire has replaced the marrow in my bones. My moods are unpredictable. I've been afraid I'll lash at Cole and he doesn't deserve my fury. Maybe with some time alone my moods will even out. Maybe it will be a good reset for both of us. I clean up my place and feel excited about getting more practice being sober.

Ain't Misbehavin'

I told Cole that if I stayed, I'd get a job to help defray the costs. I call Odell and tell her I'm looking for work and she has an idea and will pick me up in an hour.

She won't tell me where we're going, and I enjoy the mystery. As Odell drives, we catch up. We pull into a nearly empty parking lot of a brick building with very few windows. Odell makes a call and says, "We're here." The door near the end of the building opens. Odell gets out of the car and I follow.

"Zella this is Sylvia. The woman I told you about," Odell says.

Zella smiles, speaking with a silvery accent, "I understand you might be looking for a job soon. Come on in and join the party."

I walk in tentatively, last in line. We pass through a second set of doors and I hear the racket of about thirty barking dogs. Oh no, they want me to adopt a cat. I turn around and head toward the door.

"It's not what you think. Come on. Follow us," Odell says and slips her arm in mine.

As we walk between hurricane fence cages, I hear, "Hey, do you know 'Ain't Misbehavin'"? Would you sing it for it me? I love that song." I look at one dog in particular I think asked the question, and he adds, "Please, it's been so long since I've heard it."

Am I having an auditory hallucination, or have I gone bananas? Maybe I overheard a movie playing somewhere. I breathe, slow and steady, and unclench my jaw and shoulders as much as possible.

Just in case I'm not hallucinating, I mumble toward the dog, "I can't sing."

Zella and Odell keep walking. I'm relieved they didn't hear me. My fragile psyche can't take the ridicule right now.

We come to the middle of the building with a counter to our left and three offices to our right. Through a large glass door, I see the cats have the other side of the building. My heart lurches. I don't want to look, but I do. They have several scratching posts and ledges for the cats. My heart falls into my stomach. I miss Maddy. I grab my shirt and twist it hard enough to hurt.

We sit down on rickety metal chairs near a dented metal desk in one of the offices. I release my shirt and see it's wrinkled. No one says anything.

"As you can see, we don't have a large budget," says Zella who looks directly into my eyes.

"What budget?" asks Odell and they both laugh.

"We need someone to help pet the cats and walk the dogs. Odell says you're good with animals and need a job."

"That sounds amazing, but do you know I'm newly sober?"

"I know all about it. You'll be fine here," Zella insists.

I look at Odell, outraged she'd share my personal information. She shrugs.

"It's a good job," interrupts Zella, "but it does not pay very well. We do, however, offer medical benefits."

"Thank you, both of you. I haven't told Odell yet but I'm thinking about contacting an old client about more work." I hadn't thought of asking my old client for work until just now. I have my computer and can work from home and not have to think about leaving Maddy. "I'm sorry to have wasted your time," I add.

"I see. Give it some thought anyway. Maybe you'll change your mind. I understand you'd like your husband to live here, too. There might be a job opening up soon that he might be perfect for. We're poor and sometimes the work is heartbreaking, but we have big hearts and enjoy each other's company."

"I would love to work here. I'd love Cole to work here. I'll talk to him and let you know."

"I hope you change your mind. It was lovely to meet you, Sylvia." I love how Zella says my name.

She walks us to the door where we entered. As the door begins to shut, she asks, "Do you know the words to 'Ain't Misbehavin'? I love Fats Waller."

My mouth hangs open and I wonder what's going on. Was it a trick?

"You didn't know you could talk to the animals?" asks Odell when we get in the car.

I roll my eyes at her, but I wonder. I want to talk about it but instead I say, "The world has gone mad. Everything is upside down."

"Don't you love it when that happens?" Odell says.

Full-on Integrity?

Odell drops me off at my place. I sit on the couch and think. I need to make enough money to replenish what we spent on this trip. Despite an insistent tug to work at the animal shelter, it doesn't pay enough. I think about my former client and consider calling.

Around three years ago, I'd been to several weekend workshops to study a self-help technique. After the certification course ended, the developer said he had to shut down the training since in-person attendance had dropped off. I suggested putting the training online and the first task would be whipping the muddled study manual into shape. Once the manual was complete, I had everything ready to put the course online, but I'd quit for the move overseas. I decide to call the developer, which makes my stomach do backflips, so I make a junk food run to the nearest gas station.

After eating some chips and cupcakes, I feel more nauseous than nervous and make the call. I tell him my plans have changed and ask if he wants me to complete the training. He says yes and I'm suddenly employed. I hum the song, "Ain't Misbehavin'", and I remember the job at the shelter, but I don't want to think about it, so I jump online and update the software I'll need.

This project brings together all my skills. I have so many marketing ideas, but I'll keep those for later. I have the know-how to put the program online and I'll sketch out a quick five-year marketing plan for success that will turn this company into a household name. I won't have much time to write in my journal but that's okay. I'm excited and ready to get to work.

—⁓—

A month has flown by and I've gotten a lot done. I'm skipping recovery meetings for now and not calling Odell until I get an idea of how long this project will take. They hired an office manager to coordinate the project, which should give me more time for actual production. I'm hoping I'll have to attend less meetings with the developer, his wife, and two staff members. We spend a lot of time in meetings. Meetings take away from the time I could be working. The new office manager seems more than willing to sit through meeting after meeting.

The office manager and I talk by phone or video chat and go over things a few times a day. Sometimes she sounds ashy and unsure and asks me what to say to the developer. Other times she gets bossy and impatient, and her tone turns gruff and gravelly. On video, I can only see her from the chest up and her older computer camera exaggerates her features, which makes her look like she'd feel more at home attending a boxing match than at a suburban office building. She gossips and wants to give me the low down about what's happening at the office. I cringe when she gossips.

Today I finally tell her, "I don't like gossip. Please, please stop."

She says, "I don't do that anymore," and quickly adds, "but let me just tell you this one thing," and proceeds with the latest scuttlebutt.

I don't have the nerve to hang up. The developer told me she has, "full-on integrity." I'm not so sure I agree, but he's sold a lot of self-development books and probably knows best. Maybe she's different around him. Her lack of experience working in an office becomes more apparent each day. I get an awful feeling in my stomach whenever we speak.

I've got too much to do to think about it anyway. We have a tight deadline. I have to squeeze about a year's work into a few months. I see my notebook sticking out from beneath the couch where I do most of my work. I think about writing to Cave Woman and asking about the office manager. Then I look at my computer screen and push the notebook under the couch with my heel and get back to work.

Cole and I talk a few times a day. Mostly about how much work we have to get done. I wonder if he wants me to come back and live with him again, but I'm too busy to ask or maybe too afraid of what he might say.

—⟨⟩—

Five weeks into the project and I'm not sure if I'll finish on time. The work is overwhelming but a good distraction after Cole's departure. I work straight through evenings and weekends. I eat sandwiches and chips and guzzle iced tea. I'm guessing Cave Woman wouldn't approve of my diet or the long hours. I'm too busy to ask right now.

I hear people in the pool occasionally, but I only like to swim alone so I keep working.

Each day this week, I've asked the office manager not to tell me more gossip. Each time she says okay and then proceeds to gossip.

—⟨⟩—

Today—I'm not sure what day of the week it is—I'm dizzy and nauseous from so much time sitting and intensely focusing on the computer screen. In the past, I would have masked symptoms like these with alcohol. I wonder if I could drink until the project is finished and then quit again. Could I quit again? I'm not sure.

—⟨⟩—

The dizziness and nausea eased after I first quit drinking. Of course, I wasn't on the computer much. But now, the wooziness has returned, and it feels like I'm constantly on a merry-go-round with the occasional sudden trip on a Tilt-A-Whirl. I'm sure the symptoms have ramped up because I'm working on the computer so much, but I wonder if there are other contributing factors.

I order a pizza again. Trips to the grocery store take time away from work. I eat one piece but put the rest aside and work through the evening.

Around eleven p.m., I try to sleep, even though I'm barely sleeping these days.

After a few hours' sleep, I wake up to a shaking bed. I look around to see what else was shaking, thinking it was an earthquake. Nothing else moves and I quickly realize that I'm the one shaking the bed. Must be more trauma release. At least I hope so. I have absolutely no time to see a doctor.

For the past month, I've been training the new office manager to run the online platform for when we go live. She's never even made a conference call, so the learning curve is steep. I probably should be charging them for the training time. Juggling the training and my workload feels crazy.

During our training session today, she surprises me by saying, "You're at a disadvantage not being here in person. I'm going to use that."

I laugh, assume she's joking, and say, "Use it for what?" I feel like my head is wrapped in gauze and it's getting tighter by the second. I'm confused, like I'm slipping away.

"To get rid of you so I can keep this job," she whispers, I guess so no else in the office can hear her.

"That makes no sense. I'm a freelancer. I'll be gone soon anyway," I say as it dawns on me that she's serious and needs someone to blame for her inexperience. After all the help I've given her, I feel as though I've been punched in the gut. My ears ring and I feel far away, like I'm watching myself from outside the window.

"I'm just kidding," she says with no mirth.

I've heard that all my life from my dad. I deeply suspect she's not kidding.

"You may be gone sooner than you think," she suggests.

"Who will finish the work?" I ask.

"Doesn't matter. I'll take credit..." Her tone suddenly changes to light and friendly and she says, "Ok, Sil. Talk to you tomorrow. Thanks again for all your amazing work. We love you and our hearts are so filled with gratitude for you." And then she hangs up. I assume someone walked into the room for her tone to change so abruptly.

I can't quite grasp the mind games playing out here. My stomach clenches and my head spins. A familiar feeling of betrayal seizes my throat, and I feel jolted awake.

Wait a damn minute. I stand up. She can't do my job. This is absurd. I don't have time to handle their problem employees. The owners will find out about her duplicity soon enough. I'll leave it to them to figure out. Maybe I won't need to meet with the office manager so often.

After a restless night, I wake up to a hot apartment. The weather is heating up. I've been warned it gets uncomfortably hot in the summer, but I'm not sure it's even spring yet.

I start thinking about all the times over the past month or so that the office manager has lied and gossiped. She invented an affair between her and the developer and seems to like torturing me with the lurid details. Gossip divides people and makes them mistrust each other. I've never had time for that. I see her game now and I don't want to play anymore.

For the first time, when she calls today, I don't answer. She texts and promises she'll only talk about work. I call her and say, "I'll end any conversation once you start lying or gossiping. We stick to business or I hang up."

"You can't stop me. He likes me and he doesn't like you at all. He and his wife may be in business together, but they fight all the time. He told me I'll be getting a share of the profits soon. We're also writing a book together."

I hang up and feel like I can't take a deep breath. I'll have to ignore her as best as I can.

A few days later, a man I'd had some friendly conversations with during the training calls me and says he'll no longer speak with me because of the way I treat the office manager.

Why call someone to say you won't talk with her anymore? I don't understand.

Wait, I get it. I told her I wouldn't talk with her if she lied or gossiped. She's telling people I'm refusing to talk to her at all. I attempt to explain to the gentleman on the phone, but he angrily talks over me and says I shouldn't be implying there are problems between the developer and his wife.

This is bad. The office manager is telling people I'm doing the rotten things she's doing. Why does this work?

My head aches and my heart pounds, I peel my sticky legs from the plastic-covered couch and turn up the air conditioner. I have to concentrate on my deadline. I work until no other thought enters my mind.

Two days later, the office manager calls to tell me I'm not invited to any marketing meetings. How odd. I recently asked her to schedule an appointment with the developer and his wife to go over the five-year plan I'd written. She said they're not interested in talking with me, but she'd read it if I emailed it to her now. I don't think that's a good idea. I'll deal with that later. I have important work to complete and a million loose ends to tie up.

—◊—

After two and a half months I'm on a video call and I'm finally able to announce that I've finished the job. I'm shocked when the office manager says I can't tell the owners. Apparently, the other person in the office hasn't finished his portion of the project and we have to cover for him.

He pops into screen, leans over the office manager's shoulder, and tells me I'm handy to have around because they can blame me for anything that goes wrong in the office.

The cruelty should shock me more, but I don't feel much. My ears ring and my head vibrates like a rung bell. The worst part of working for yourself is still having to deal with people. I feel like I'm in sixth grade again and dealing with a bully. I need to quit and get away from these mind games. Or at least find some support.

I grab my phone and nervously call the owner and tell him I think his new office manager is lying. He says, "I know she's lying but she has a great work ethic."

I want to say, *Isn't truthfulness a big part of ethics?* but before I can say anything, he adds, "I've been hearing about your behavior during this time and I'm not pleased."

What behavior? My tongue goes numb, and the numbness feels like it's spreading to my brain. It hits me like an electrical shock that I've been the victim of a smear campaign. I can't speak, so he does.

He tells me to keep working but not to speak about any of this with his wife.

Especially the lying part.

I stare at my phone in disbelief and hang up. I put my laptop aside and wonder how many sankes will cut my legs off before I learn to recognize the sound of their chainsaws approaching. I'm gutted, confused, and furious. I slide to the floor. My head spins and I squeeze the carpet between my fingers. The room spins at what feels like 100 mph. I don't know why but I yell, "All is well," over and over until the spinning subsides. It lasts only a few minutes, but no matter how much I shout, I know one thing for sure: All is not well.

I can't remember the last time I left the apartment. When did I last go for a swim?

When did I last go to a meeting?

All I've done for the past few months is endlessly move videos, photos, text, and graphics around my computer screen, creating a project for people who are attacking me. But I can't stop. I feel compelled to get back to work, so I pull myself off the floor.

While looking at the computer, my center vision suddenly drops away. Panic thunders through my heart hard enough that I feel it pounding in my hands and feet. I know this isn't good. I've lost the ability to deal with what is right in front of me. Or rather, what's not right in front of me. I'm not dead so maybe I'm okay. The best thing to do is get this job over with and move on. That's a good idea. Now that I've decided to finish, I bet I'll regain my full vision any minute now. If I move my computer to my side, I can see out of the corner of my eye and still work.

I try typing a few words, but my hands become numb and I physically can't continue working. I hold the phone up to the side of my eye to find Cole in my contacts. When he answers, only about every fifth word comes out of my mouth. He probably thinks I'm drunk.

I shout, "Not drunk," and then, "Help," and, "Need doc."

Even though Cole is in the north, he tells me to walk to the front office, that he'll call me a cab and tell them to take me to the hospital. I try to stay on the sidewalk but keep stumbling into the grass. By the time I get to the front office, the cab has already arrived. I don't think about much of anything. The bright sunlight washes out most of the landscape and it looks like a whiteout. Is it snowing?

How did I get back north? I attempt to remember but my mind gives me nothing.

An attendant helps me out of the cab and into a wheelchair. He is so nice that I want to hug him.

I arrive at the front desk and cock my head sideways so I can see the nurse. I point to my mouth and shake my head no. I move my hands up and down in front of my face and point to my eyes and shake my head no. She says, "You can't speak or see in front of you?" I nod yes. Before I can take another breath, three nurses surround me, one on either side and one behind me. Uh-oh, this ain't good.

She shouts, "Don't worry now, ok? But we're putting you in stroke protocol just to be on the safe side. But promise me you won't worry, ok?"

I hadn't even considered a stroke. Oh no, I'm having a stroke. I feel faint and the lower part of my face goes numb. I'm now having a panic attack as well.

They lead me to an exam room and another nurse shouts, "You're in what's called 'stroke protocol.'"

I try to say I can hear fine, but nothing comes out of my mouth. I cover my ears because her shouting hurts. I've had a lot of times in my life where I didn't know what to say, when I stammered and mumbled, but I've never experienced an outright inability to say anything at all. Fear rushes through my head, chest, and stomach like a cloudburst. My heart pounds so hard I feel the veins in my neck jumping.

I've rebelled against the idea that life should be all work and no play. I never once suspected in all my life I'd die from overwork and being stabbed in the back over a damn job. I'd be furious if I wasn't so confused.

"We'll be monitoring you until the doctor arrives and then take you in for a CT scan. All this needs to happen in a ten-minute window. Do you have health insurance?"

I attempt to say, "In another state. Does that count?" but the words sit stubbornly in my mind. I can still see out of the side of my eyes and I move my head around until I spot my small backpack and point. She hands it to me, and I root around and find my wallet. I keep the insurance card behind a plastic window. I hold it up to the side of my head to make sure it's the right card. I hand the card to the nurse.

The nurse with my insurance card leaves the room and the other takes my blood pressure again and says, "It's very high. Higher than it was when you came in."

I try to mumble, "No shit," but I just shake my head yes and then no and shrug my shoulders. If they need me to diagnose myself, what are all these machines for?

By the time the nurse with the insurance card returns, the ten-minute stroke protocol window has long passed. She said it wouldn't cover the visit. "Can you afford to pay?"

I nod yes and point to my wallet and feel for the part of my wallet that holds my credit cards.

"Can I take it?"

What choice do I have? I nod yes.

Again, the nurse leaves to check my credit card. The other nurse said if my credit card is good, they'd be charging me every time my bill hit $10,000. "Do you agree to that?" she asks.

The anger wakes me up as if a fairy godmother has zapped me with her magic wand.

I can see better and the panic attack is clearing. I say, "Doc firth."

Just then a doctor walks in. I want to say, "I will not agree to unlimited access to my credit card until I have some idea of what is happening to me," but instead I say, "What wrong wit me? Money not now."

She looks at the nurses and then looks at me. I feel the heat of anger in my face. She asks the nurses to leave the room. After looking in my eyes and listening to my heart, she sighs and says, "I'm sorry for the delay. There are most likely two explanations. It might be a stoke or it might be a migraine."

When I speak, some words are clear and some I lose, but she seems to understand well enough. "On 'puter all time. Is mmmmmm." I add, "Stroke widow passsss…"

"I know," she offers but doesn't apologize. Maybe she's tired of apologizing. "I can't in good conscience let you go without a CT scan. Okay?"

I nod because if I speak, I'll shout, "NO!" and it probably is best to know. At least I won't have to guess whether it was a migraine or a stroke.

Five hours and $15,000 later, the doctor says the veins in my head are "beautiful" with no sign of a stroke. I can leave. The doctor told me the migraine was probably from too much time on electronic devices. She prescribes medication to keep it from happening again.

Good. I need to get back to work.

Chapter 20

Skydiving

I text Cole to tell him what happened and how much it cost. He texts back that the only important thing is that I'm okay. I wonder how he really feels and bite back tears.

My vision is clear by the time I head back to my place with a bag full of drugs from the hospital pharmacy and strict orders to stay off all electronics. I give the taxi driver a twenty-dollar bill because I can't remember paying the first cab driver. I tell him to keep the change. I pass the mess in the living room, close the curtain in front of the sliding glass door in the bedroom, and lay down. I look at the medications. I have to call Odell to let her know what I'll be taking. Will she even talk to me since I stopped calling and going to meetings? I'm not sure but there's something I have to do first.

Dear Cave Woman,

I worked until I was sick and got gaslighted for my efforts. I spent more money in five hours in the emergency room than I made putting this project together. I'm scared, I'm hurt, and worried I may never work on a computer again. Can you help?

Why haven't you been asking me about this job all along? I could have guided you.

Now, it's too late.

Please don't tell me that. Too late for what?

To have made better choices. To have followed your intuition. To have asked for my guidance before choosing a job.

But I—

And why have you been working around the clock? No one else is.

You're right. I was afraid to stop working. If I stopped, I would have realized I was carrying the whole load, including all the blame. I don't want to think about it. I just wanted to keep working. Isn't that awful? Please forgive me. Please. I'm so sorry.

You've substituted alcohol for work. Neither of which can shut out the truth forever. You've turned away from the healthy community you need, inside and out.

You're hurting yourself and your future.

I'm back with you to stay. Okay?

Good. I wanted to hear you say it.

But none of this had to happen. Why do people think cruelty is an effective way to manage a business? I've seen this so many times.

Bullies and sankes cause enormous pain. Corporations often promote and take on the characteristics of sankes.

Bullies call cruelty being "tough" by claiming they're protecting the best interests of the company or their families.

Sankes make themselves seem like victims while simultaneously destroying and victimizing innocent people, resulting in staggering damage.

What can I do?

Let yourself feel the anger, so you don't become its prisoner, so the denial of your intuition doesn't land you in the emergency room again, so you can rebuild even stronger boundaries. So you don't become cruel, too.

How do I make this job work? It's perfect for me.

That's your betrayed inner cave person speaking. Workaholism keeps you from dealing with the truth, just like alcohol.

Working obsessively was another way to ignore emotions? Another way to obey the old script and the self-pressure it causes?

You had a chance to turn this around before you brushed aside the job at the animal shelter without consulting me. You had another chance to turn this around when you had an awful feeling about the office manager. Or when she wouldn't stop gossiping and the owner defended her gaslighting. You overrode your gut sense and lost sight of your own safety.

I thought the problem would take care of itself. I thought I was doing the right thing by letting them deal with their own employees.

You let the gaslighting continue, which made you part of the problem.

I see that now. I remained silent. I worked such long hours I not only lost myself, I lost my eyesight. I wound up blind and mute and in the emergency room.

You were blinded by betrayal. All the adrenaline from the 3F Red Zone became so overwhelming, your body raged up a storm. What you experienced was in direct opposition to the values you thought the company stood for. You ignored the warning signs and your brilliant body acted to warn you.

My body literally won't let me torture myself. It rebelled to save me. I didn't speak up for myself, so I became mute. I ignored the truth and lost part of my sight. I wasn't being heard and I lost the ability to speak. I didn't call out the hypocrisy and I lost the self-worth I was beginning to pick up. It'd be nice to notice the subtler clues, so my body doesn't have to go to such extremes. Are bodily symptoms always this literal?

No, symptoms don't often fit so easily into an analogy. Wanting to speak up for yourself and the impulse to get the job done created a profound contradiction. You sat hunched over your computer and ignored your body's survival urge to fight or flee an unhealthy situation.

I ignored the warning signs by working obsessively?

Yes, you ignored the subtler signs by pushing past your physical capacity and continued working. The symptoms could've ramped up in any number of different ways.

Warning signs don't go away, they get louder.

Tune in daily to my inner hive and write to you?

Absolutely. You would've seen the storm brewing and gotten the hell out of the way.

I witnessed a lot of meanness, but I wasn't being physically attacked.

Your Survival Brain responds to any attack; physical or psychological.

What do I do?

What does your body want to do?

—⚍—

I spiral my hands and feet and feel my hips and shoulders to get more in my body. What do you want right now, body?

—⚍—

Dear Cave Woman,

That's odd. My body wants to skydive. What a surprising and terrible idea for my head.

No, listen to your body. This is good advice. Put your body in a skydiving position.

—⏣—

I roll over on my belly and lift my arms and legs and sway slightly from side to side as if I'm maintaining my balance in midair. My shoulder blades move toward my spine, giving my upper back muscles a nice massage. I lay flat and rest my head in the crook of my arm and my whole body sighs.

I wake up a few hours later.

It's 3:33 a.m. I throw out some pizza boxes and empty iced tea bottles. I turn on my computer long enough to send an email telling the developer I need to take few weeks of sick leave. I shut down my computer and throw dirty clothes into a pile for laundry. It feels satisfying to move, to sing in the shower, and to see clearly. It feels miraculous to only think about questions I have for Cave Woman.

—⏣—

Dear Cave Woman,

Why did my body like that position? On my belly, like I was skydiving?

Because it was the opposite of hunching over your computer. You helped your mind and body know you'd chosen to get out of harm's way.

If I'd spoken up during this awful job, maybe things could have been different.

No, things wouldn't have been different. Part of you

made a choice to get away. **If you'd written to me, you'd have known sooner. But part of you made a choice not to create more unjust chaos. You could have fought at any point, but you knew you'd lose the tiny ripple of serenity you'd gained in recovery. Unconsciously, you knew jumping further into the fray would not have served your sobriety.**

I knew I couldn't win?

You knew you didn't want to win. Not for this for job, not for these people.

And if I stay?

If you continue working for this company, you'll be a hypo-crite, too. Like the developer. Like the office manager.

Well, hell, I suppose we're all hypocrites. But I can make a different choice not to add to, as you said, the unjust chaos. I can still feel the grip of addiction, the pull to keep working despite all the cruelty.

Your body speaks the truth. Are you willing to listen?

It's all so unfair. Cruelty wins again. I'll have to look for another job. I may not be able to work on a computer again. And cruel people get away with everything. And nothing happens to them. How did humanity get to this place?

When humans stopped living in a healthy community, where cooperation and equity were an absolute necessity, they lost a great deal of common sense and decency.

There's no justice. People kowtow to the cruel. Do people only get ahead because they're willing to bulldoze over others? What's wrong with the world?

Cruelty and abuse signal that something is wrong and the culture needs to heal longstanding wounds. No one wins when people control and manipulate others. No one, not even the perceived "winners."

This feels so hopeless.

In my time, we knew something was wrong with the whole community when individuals acted out.

So, the individual isn't responsible for their actions because it's a societal issue?

Individuals contribute to healing the community by healing themselves, including their own insecurities, cruelties, and addictions. Hopelessness will lessen when you can notice your inner cave child is in charge. When you can see different options, you'll know it's possible for the entire world. Your capacity to heal yourself is so much greater than you know, but you can't force someone else to heal.

Should I feel sorry for the office manager? What if her childhood was super messed up?

No need to feel sorry for sankes, they're not destructive and devious as a result of childhood abuse. If all sankes came from childhood abuse, they would outnumber everyone else. And either way, experiencing abuse does not give one license to abuse others.

But what about competition? I've seen competition ruin entire companies. As a freelancer, I've worked on many projects for loads of companies and the one thing that limits success is deception and backstabbing within the team. If the team collaborates with an "all for one and one for all" mindset, the chances of success skyrocket.

You're right, cooperation increases innovation and profits exponentially.

When I explain this to a team I'm freelancing for, I'm met with reassurances that everyone's on board. And then the backstabbing starts. The backstabbers win a lot of the time, and they're usually the people with the least amount of experience and creativity.

Betraying others in order to succeed creates more destruction. Undue competition is its own worst reward. Competition leads to additional meanness, hurt, havoc, and disconnection. Every hurt,

every injustice, always comes back to lack of empathy and ignorance about the best ways to create easeful, cooperative success.

Success can be easy and doesn't have to include deception? If
that's true, it's a deeply buried secret.

**Anything built on betrayal is unstable. You live in a very
unstable society.**

Why don't people want to work together as a team?

**Because many modern people are stuck in the scarcity of
the Dividing Mind without any counterbalancing skills. I'll
teach you an emotion counterbalancing skill when you're
feeling less distracted and rattled.**

Okay, but how would companies know who was the betrayer
and who was the betrayed if the perpetrator is lying?

**Who's getting the work done? Those who can deliver the
final product don't need to lie about their work or betray their
colleagues. Their work speaks for itself. Or should.**

We've lost so much since your time.

**Humans working together, living and loving in symbiotic
connection, has been a tragic loss. My community mimicked
nature in all its mutable glory. We lived a life of delicate rich-
ness, awestruck and engaged.**

You stole all your best ideas from nature?

Of course, we knew our true teachers.

Modern people believe competition is everything.

**People crave connection from the moment they're born.
Sadly, people believe that deceiving others is the only way to
feel safe. Deception only creates more danger. Every betrayal
pulls humans away from solidarity and contentment. Cruel people may find monetary success, but they will never feel secure
or joyful. They'll spend their entire lives jumping between jus-
tification and shallow excitement, chasing the high of the scam**

or running from the shame kindled by their deceptions.

Competition is so unfair and has broken my heart. Again.

Your world needs broken-hearted people who are committed to regaining wholeness no matter how wide the cracks. You're letting your heart break to recover your wholeness.

I feel like I lost my last chance to use all my skills at one job.

You've played below the radar for a long time. You thought it would keep you safe. You blindly, and without my guidance, stuck your neck out and it got nicked. Come back to me and the work we started together. Imagine what we can do together. Each day of recovery will contain unexpected successes.

My brain is working very slowly. I may need you to repeat things a few hundred times. Can you remind me where we were?

By all means.

Keep questioning social norms and noticing the Unreliable Narrator.

Meet feelings and survival sensations with validation and understanding.

Return to your sober friends and enjoy some community.

Don't forget others struggle, too.

Call on me. I'm available night and day.

Staying Hidden

I eat some leftover miso soup from the refrigerator. It's too late to call Odell so I take my meds and get in bed. I sleep but wake up before dawn. I remember this empty feeling from my first sober days. I want to jump on my computer and start working again. I have two weeks to decide whether to return or resign. I attempt to go back to sleep but every time I close my eyes, I see the image of a bear. I'm panicking and need help. I feel trapped like I'm wedged inside a pile of boulders.

—⚍—

Dear Cave Woman,

I feel helpless. I'll never feel well again. My head feels like it did when I was hungover; dense and squirrelly. I'm nauseous and hungry at the same time. There isn't a meeting for another three hours. Each time I close my eyes, I see a bear. I'm confused. Am I losing my mind? In all seriousness, I think I need to go back to drinking.

That's your protective Mama bear. She's helping you heal while you repair your hive.

What can I do? How can I help myself heal? Can I change my Survival Brain by meditating?

Do you have twenty years to spare?

Very funny. No, I do not.

In a way, you already do meditate by focusing on every possible danger. You're focused on worry. Also, meditating on the chatter of the Unreliable Narrator keeps you frozen and vulnerable to victimization.

So, I shouldn't meditate?

Wait until you can soothe your own nervous system or find a guided meditation you like. You could also take a few minutes to drift aimlessly. Take a break from improving yourself. And remember that Spare Tire breathing, among other things, helps regulate your nervous system, giving you the benefits of meditation.

Why aren't the Survival Brain patterns on my side?

Again, they are, but the patterns that protected you ear-lier in your life are not necessarily the ones you want leading you as an adult.

For example?

For example, one of your patterns is to stay hidden. As a child, staying hidden helped keep you safe from some of your father's sabotage. As an adult, staying hidden makes it tough to have your efforts recognized. Friends, family, and employ-ers become suspicious if you hide most of the time.

I still have a hard time remembering that what my mind tells me isn't always accurate.

You remembered just now. Very good, my little cub.

Can I change my mind by repeating affirmations and inten-tions?

Not if you're attempting to bypass your emotions. Neither your body nor your emotions are deceived by platitudes. Also, affirmations and intentions might add too much pressure at this stage in your recovery.

Do you have a magic spell I can repeat?

Let me think. The Inner Narrator was meant to keep you safe and reassured. To rewrite the tapes of the Unreliable Nar-rator, let's use some assurances. Try these: It's safe to feel what I'm feeling; it's safe for me to take a few Spare Tire Breaths; it's natural to not always feel well as I heal; it's safe to let my mind wander; it's safe to daydream; it's safe to be rebellious; it's safe to rest while my body relearns to sleep naturally; it's safe to drop the constrictions in my shoulders and jaw.

I like assurances. I feel less squirrelly. What's next?

Exercise your imagination. Bring the heat of your emo-tions to your daydreams until the scene feels real.

I did that the other day. I imagined living in a seaside town.

When I opened my eyes and looked out the window, I fully expected to see an ocean view instead of the local park.

Sparks ignited by vivid daydreams light up new shortcuts in your brain, which escorts out the old and invites intuitive insights.

I imagined walking toward the beach. I could smell the briny sea and see the waves. I could hear the sand crunching and hissing under my flip flops. I felt elated.

And, by daydreaming, you moved your focus away from the business of the Survival Brain. Your body could rest and relearn how to play.

Weren't you always focused on survival?

Not at all. When I became separated from my community, I did focus more on my Survival Brain. My protective worries would rise. I felt the constant danger that you tend to focus on. While profoundly uncomfortable, I knew it would guide me safely back to my community.

Focusing on danger, when you're not in serious trouble, feels awful. When you consistently focus on danger, a lot of adrenaline courses through your body that doesn't get utilized.

Should I do yoga?

Yoga can be helpful if it's something you enjoy. Yoga was devised for people who sat in meditation all day to wring out emotions that lived deep in the tissues.

Before I left the frozen north, I did a seven-minute yoga routine each morning for a year. It wore me out. Is that pathetic or what?

The consistency, not the time spent practicing, benefits you now. Lasting change starts with small steps.

I cried each time I did yoga. Now, do you think it's pathetic?

Not at all. I think you got a head start on feeling your body and moving your emotions.

What else can I do?

Dancing and singing help.

I can't dance or sing.

Okay, we'll save those for later.

What else?

You can learn to appreciate old patterns you no longer need, such as staying hidden. Appreciate how staying hidden kept you safe in the same way you imagined living near the ocean.

You're joking, right? That sounds downright masochistic. But I do recognize staying hidden as a pattern. Staying hidden can feel cozy for half a second, but mostly it feels infuriating, lonely, and downright paralyzing. What's to appreciate?

The love.

You want me to love feeling infuriated?

Yes. All emotions are contained in love, even anger.

I don't understand.

When you feel love, you're feeling your emotions in flow with each other.

Love staying hidden and all the emotions that helped keep it in place?

By all means. Love staying hidden's bravery and strength. Appreciate the agony and the bittersweet drama staying hidden created to keep you well-concealed.

Love staying hidden for all it has done for you.

I started hiding after I broke my leg. I think I was eight years old and stuck inside the house.

Yes, and you were very active before that. You stayed active and kept breaking your cast, which forced you to keep still.

As a kid, you moved out painful energy by exploring the

woods, tossing water balloons, and riding your bike. You lost that when you had to keep still.

I remember. And I became cautious after getting the cast off.

You started looking for other ways to move energy, which led you to addictive patterns.

All from a broken leg?

From not understanding how to help emotional energy flow.

How do I let staying hidden know I don't need it anymore?

Staying hidden is a crucial skill to have. All animals, at times, need to stay hidden. For you, staying hidden happens whether you want it to or not. That's what you want to change.

Write to me from the viewpoint of staying hidden and all its achievements.

Okay, here goes.

I am safely hidden, and I am so proud of all that I have achieved.

I fear that without me, Sylvia would have gotten an office job she hated and thrown herself off the Brooklyn Bridge.

I fear that Sylvia would have become more and more careless without me, which would have been very dangerous living and drinking alone in a city.

I fear that without me, she would have killed her father for abusing her mother. I helped her stay stuck and close to home, too drunk or hungover to act.

I want to stop. This is kind of weird and intense. Is that enough?

Of course. Can you see how brilliantly staying hidden did its job? Can you feel the intensity like you felt the seaside town?

Yes, I'm on its side. Staying hidden is a fighter and a renegade.

Yes, by your side. Not in control or in charge.

Okay, what other pattern needs loosening? I'm ready to see habitual patterns from a new vantage point. I feel like I have a new set of spark plugs. But wait. I suddenly feel angry. Ragefully angry. I feel angry that I didn't get to choose so much of what I experienced. I'm angry I wasn't taught I had a choice. I hate how much shame I'm left with because I didn't know we were robots ruled by outdated information.

As more patterns shift, you won't feel so robotic.

But what do I do with all this anger?

Feel anger's electrical current surging through your body, cleaning up the remnants from staying hidden so long. Feel the power of your own revolution. Feel the powerful surge anger gives to your immune system.

I'm angry I let the world get the better of me. Can I ever forgive myself?

Love the little match girl inside you who felt rejected and invisible and used all her matches to light the way for others but forgot to leave any fire for herself. Love the pathetic bedraggled pauper, love the power of defiance, love the mulish stubbornness, like a wrongly accused criminal who'd rather remain in jail than plead guilty.

I see how staying hidden did its job exceptionally well and how the anger helps. Can I appreciate other emotions, like anger, with fear, with sorrow?

Absolutely. Appreciation isn't just for happy feelings. Appreciate the heartbreak, the cringe-worthy tragedies, the loneliness, and all the loss. Appreciate how addiction brought you a compassionate view of humanity that non-addicts rarely see.

This is how you transform.

I feel a wave of powerful, angry appreciation like it's propelling me forward.

And the helpless feeling passed?

It did. And I have absolutely no craving to drink.

Good. You're learning to speak to emotions with emotions. It's a form of communication all animals except modern humans speak fluently. As you allow the back and forth between your mind and body, your muscles won't have to strain to shield you.

You'll enter the 3F Red Zone less often.

How will I know I've mastered this skill?

When the patterns you've judged as wrong receive validation, you'll feel the change physically, like a deep belly laugh or like a heavy burden has been lifted. Emotions are chemical; attention to them alchemical.

Then the next pattern that's no longer useful will emerge?

When another stuck pattern is ready to be discharged, open your arms and embrace the sensations. Appreciate them all, and you'll walk the rest of your life hand-in-hand with your health-giving Mama bear, half-bathed with incandescent wit, lighting up the hidden shadows of your mind.

Urgency

I wake up around 9:00 a.m. and call Odell. She's been up for hours, which I should have guessed.

"I wondered if I'd ever hear from you again," Odell says before I even say hello.

"I've been working. A lot. I worked so much I got an ocular migraine," I say.

"I bet you wish you'd taken the job at the animal shelter," Odell states.

"No kidding. I spent more on a visit to the ER than I made. I thought the animal shelter paid too little, but I would have made more money in the end," I admit.

"Did you drink?" Odell asks.

"I'm in a world of hurt, but I didn't drink. I think I may have developed a bit of a work addiction."

"That can happen. Want to go to a meeting?" Odell asks.

"Yes, please. But I can't drive."

"I'm offering. I'll pick you up in an hour."

"That would be amazing. Thank you."

"Don't thank me yet. You have a lot of work ahead."

"I guessed as much," I say. We hang up, and I shower and get dressed.

Old Movies

After the meeting, Odell takes me to a health food market, and we each buy some groceries. By the time she drops me off at my place, I'm very tired. I told Odell what had happened, but I'm still not able to speak well. I stumbled over words and forgot what I was saying half the time. Odell looked concerned. I zoned out during the meeting, too, but it felt good to be back.

Odell offers to sit by my bed while I rest, but I turn her down.

"What a nice offer," I say and zone out again.

She nods in understanding, and I take my groceries and leave the car.

I put my bags on the counter and grab the remote. I feel like watching an old movie like I did with my mom.

After the third movie, I go to bed and wake up at 2:00 a.m. I peel and eat an orange and wash my hands and face very slowly. The water feels good. I get back in bed but pull my notebook and pen from the bedside table.

—ɯ—

Dear Cave Woman,

Here we are again. Just the two of us at 2:00 a.m. I'm still recovering from my latest debacle, but I feel this urgency to do something useful in the world, despite all my failed attempts. Isn't that stupid? I want to help those who have been abused or exploited. What a joke. Everyone's just out for themselves, which makes me insane. I've felt this urgency most of my life. Make it go away.

You saw cruelty early in life. You learned about widespread injustice at a young age. You've also felt this urgency since you were little. What do all these things have in common?

Failure?

And?

Wanting to make things different?

And how do you go about—

The world is in trouble; millions are in trouble. Would someone please do something please! Help. Help. HELP! We seem more worried about clogged gutters and shiny hubcaps than each other. I've got to do something before I—

But you don't want to explode on those already in need.

I tried to help people by going to Haiti.

And what would have happened if you'd gone?

Give me a minute.

—ɯ—

I'm sitting on the ground in the middle of a narrow street. People are selling food, fabric, herbs, and spices. Open suitcases have spilled all around me. I'm blocking foot traffic. The vendors are looking at me with concern. They ask if I'm okay and I say I'm here to help. They smile sadly.

———m———

Dear Cave Woman,

I get it now. I was a wreck. The people in Haiti would have ended up taking care of me, not the other way around. I felt such urgency to help, I forgot to be useful. I would have been the one in need. I would have taken, not given. What do I do now?

Right now, you go outside and notice what you hear.

———m———

I take my notebook and open the sliding glass door that has a view of the park. I slip out on the tiny cement porch. About thirty feet away, two women sit on the ground playing acoustic guitars and singing. Maybe they couldn't sleep either. I can't pick out the tune but can hear their melodies blending. Light notes of jasmine float around me.

———m———

Dear Cave Woman,

What can I do? What do people need?

They want exactly what you wanted in a job and exactly what you need in recovery. Collaboration, to be heard, and to be believed.

What about the panic?

What can you do right now?

Talk to you, listen, learn, ask. Continue my recovery. Heal my own wounds and not bury them under the pretense of helping others.

And what do you hear?

A collaboration. A melody. Harmony. And I bet playing and singing together so beautifully took a lot of practice.

Lots and lots of practice.

Not Easily Mended

For four days, Odell has picked me up, taken me to a meeting, then to the health food store for groceries, herbal teas, and supplements.

Today, after she drops me off, I throw my keys on the small kitchen table and lay across the couch. All the time spent sitting here working like a madwoman comes back to me. Shame, like a blast of hot water, floods my veins. Anger comes back and digs at my chest like a shovel, troubling my already broken heart.

I fixate on the Unreliable Narrator who tells me I should have known better and that I'll always be inadequate.

I yell "stop" but the cycle begins again. I'm exhausted by the long process ahead.

Betrayal is not easily mended.

I feel like I've been given a respite from the Unreliable Narrator the last three days. My emotions are nudging me back to alertness. I'm not sure I'm ready.

If I stop the replay in my mind, I feel empty. I have to fill this emptiness before I do something stupid. I felt okay for a few days, almost numb, but now I'm getting moments of panic again. Cave Woman, help me, please.

—⚞—

Dear Cave Woman,

I'm still obsessed with the betrayal at this job and having moments of panic.

Considering what you've been through, I'm not surprised. You understand that your mind is in replay mode. You felt the shame and anger. That's a lot of progress without reaching for an old habit. Remember, you're new to confirming how you feel.

You'll get better with practice.

Like adding grease to the cogs of my mind-body self?

Yes, you're still a bit rusty. The work you're doing will smooth out the sharp edges. Are you worrying about the future?

Well, yeah. How many more sankes are in my future? Where will I work? You even said some workplaces mimic sankes?

They do.

Can the human race go on like this?

Not for long. Many workplaces are full of duplicity, deception, and rancor. The opposite of what we all crave as hopeful pack animals. Duplicitous workplaces engender contention instead of cooperation. Management by manipulation fosters a kill-or-be-killed mentality. Many companies and institutions claim community values of appreciation and encouragement, but it's hypocritical.

See why I'm upset? Is all the greed and deception too pervasive to fix?

I've seen the wave of greed and deception rise, and I'm

prepared to watch it crest and recede.

That's nice, but can you be more specific?

I'll do my best. Most sanke-led corporate cultures think the only way to get ahead is to have colleagues compete with and deceive each other.

They still make a lot of money. Corporations have so much money, they'll merge with governments soon.

Excessive corporate influence is a threat to democracy.

Does deception equal success?

Deception works to a certain extent but significantly limits success and erodes hope for healthy communities worldwide. Instead, corporations could bolster the health of the communities that make their wealth possible.

I'd like to succeed at something. I'm tired.

It's a monkey-see-monkey-do kind of universe. If we manipulate to gain favor, we get more experiences of needing to manipulate to gain favor. If we struggle to get work, we get the experience of struggling at work.

And when coworkers are competitive with each other, the entire company gets the experience of continued, unrelenting competition?

Yes. Very good. The result creates an endless loop of backstabbing and exhausting hard work.

But people say, "That's just the way it is. If I don't deceive and manipulate, I'll lose my job and career, and terrible things will happen."

Backstabbers don't realize terrible things are already happening and they're often the source. The larger world mirrors their actions. Eventually, sanke-led corporations become sanke-led governments. Remarkably, slight changes can produce a better outcome.

We can have good workplaces if people are willing to work

together as a healthy community?

If companies became what they pretend to be, they'd lose the self-defeating behaviors. They'd be appreciative, cooperative, encouraging. Not only would employees be spared the backstabbing, lie-for-lie scenario, they'd be happier, and companies would experience far more productivity, creativity, and success. Most importantly, they'd contribute to the larger community and no longer behave like criminal enterprises.

I hate being rejected. I hate being the one who takes the blame. I'm not a garbage dump.

Many people build themselves up by diminishing others. They know in their bones something is missing. They feel empty without a healthy community and attempt to fill it with all sorts of things, including blame and gossip. The bullying can be very subtle or quite aggressive. If bullies put their efforts into positive change, your world would be a very different place.

And sankes?

Sankes build themselves up by diminishing others and don't see a thing wrong with doing so. They often thrill at hurting others.

Does it help to know you're not alone?

It does. It helps me not take it all so personally. And all I can do is get away?

As fast as you can. And—this is important—continue to build generous and emotionally healthy communities inside and out. Continue to learn and explore what recovery could mean for every kind of human mishap and abuse.

I care so much about finding a collaborative community that I grieve every time it doesn't work out.

I know, my little water bear. Bullies, or people who use bul-

lies as a shield, are not your people. People who have been burned by bullies are very wary. Remember to look for the wary people. You can bolster each other up.

I have such longing to be part of a solution. It's physically painful.

Like everyone, you long for a healthy community, but some of your longing comes from ideas that want to be born.

Longing is the beginning of creation. And by the way, ideas don't care if they live in a museum, are written about and revered for ages, or are taped to your kitchen wall. Ideas want you to know the gleeful rush of creation. Ideas want you to enjoy the millions of years that went into making you and your clamorous ideas.

Let me tell you a story.

Medicines only comprised a small portion of our healing rituals, but many of us enjoyed the process of bringing the medicinal potions to life.

My healthy hive and I lived among riches. Trees, plants, fruits, and minerals loaned us their essence for healing and taught us perspective. We ate well. We lived well. We were rarely without food or water. Occasionally we'd ask neighboring communities to help if the land had rumbled and shook or temporarily washed away our access to Earth's abundance. The lack was always temporary and never personal. The Earth sometimes moves like a walrus shifting during sleep.

My community particularly loved making medicines. Keen on observing how animals healed themselves, we gleaned instructions on doing the same for ourselves. We'd steam, boil, and press healing from the perfusion of colorful convenience provided by Mother Earth.

One year, brimming with the herbal medicines we'd made to share as widely as possible, we packed to visit neighboring communities.

One of our young people thought we should receive something in return for the medicines we provided to our neighbors. With great excitement, they agreed to ask for fabric, teas, and dried food in exchange for our medicines.

As we finished packing, a woman who was so old she'd practically turned back into pure wisdom told us to debate this idea.

We talked and talked.

Those who were most drawn to making medicine decided we should receive the fabric, teas, and dried food in exchange.

Some argued they provided the most firewood for making medicines and deserved more goods in return.

Others who hunted and provided the fat to add to some of our medicines claimed they contributed the most.

We fought and argued for several days. At a stalemate and thoroughly stuck, we returned to the wise woman and asked her why she wanted us to fight. We blamed her for our dilemma.

She patiently asked us to remember that our neighbors already gave us fabric, teas, and dried food, in addition to lavish meals, delicate thin bones and thread for repairs, ingredients for medicines from plants and minerals not in our region, new members to add to our community, news of other communities they had visited, and stories that expanded our worldview, which she considered the greatest gift of all.

She told us that tragedies often begin when one community thinks their goods are not traded fairly. People become greedy and paranoid. They'd pillage or deny resources that used to be freely shared and cause much suffering.

Modern people also have abundance. Unfortunately, your people have been taught they must fight for limited resources, which causes people to hoard and ironically creates the lack they fear. Lack of abundance is a difficult illusion for modern people to shatter, but it must be shattered.

Lasting success requires innovation, cooperation, and a ludicrous amount of whimsy. It's fun, not dull, and lifeless, or soul-killing. Feel our camaraderie and watch it reappear.

Cave Woman's story has me thinking about Cole. I call him, and we end up talking for two hours, the longest we've spoken since my job ended. We share ideas and laugh a lot. My heart feels warm and slightly more open to what might come next.

"I'll have to stay an extra month to recover," I say.

Cole says, "You're an old pro at recovery now. You can do this, I'm certain."

"That's an excellent point. Gosh, you're smart. How did you end up with such a loser weirdo like me?"

"You're not a loser, and I like weirdos. My life would be boring without you."

"Are you sure you wouldn't prefer boring?" I dare to ask.

"I'm sure. Just get better, okay?"

Chapter 21

Buddhist Meeting

After getting back in bed last night, I listen to an audiobook online. They help me rest when I can't sleep. I wonder if I could mention at a meeting how audiobooks help me sleep. Might help someone else.

Odell is busy today, and I need a meeting. Asking strangers for rides makes me nervous. Odell said it would be good for me. I write down a script and pull out a list with phone numbers, screw up my courage, and start calling. With the first call, I get no answer. The second goes to voice mail. I feel relieved. I can tell Odell I tried, but no one answered. One more, and then I'll give up. My courage is waning. I'm about to hang up when Samron answers.

I read from the script I wrote:

"Hi, my name is Sil. I got your number from a phone list. I've been in recovery for a few months now. I'm wondering, do you have a minute?"

"I do have time. What can I help you with?" she asks.

"First, can you tell me how to say your name?"

She laughs and says, "It's pronounced like Sam plus rin, like ring without the G. Thanks for asking."

"Thanks for talking to me, Samron. I recently worked too much on my computer, and I've had eye troubles and can't drive right now. Do you happen to be going to any meetings soon?" I told her where I lived.

She said, "You're in luck, but I hope you don't mind going to a Buddhist meeting? That's where I'm headed next. Today, actually."

"I'd love to go to a Buddhist meeting. Does it matter if I'm not Buddhist?"

"Not at all. You might really like it. I do."

I told her I was looking forward to meeting her, and we arranged to meet by the front office.

Samron looks like she could hold her own in a street fight, with thick black curly hair, a knee-length black dress, a spiral silver bracelet, and a cut-off denim jacket. As a Buddhist, Samron doesn't look like what I had in mind. I love when stereotypes are shattered. After a pleasant drive and friendly conversation, we arrive at a Buddhist center.

I never would have guessed such a lovely temple with a well-kept garden held recovery meetings. For the first ten minutes, we sit in meditation. I fear I'll start to laugh, which almost makes me laugh. It would be so horrible to laugh right now, which makes me start to giggle. I cover it with a cough and a smile, then I remember to send my wild children off to play. Those mischievous devils, trying to get me in trouble. I spend the meditation imagining a little town with everything their impish hearts could desire.

"My ego just keeps getting in the way," says a Black woman in a business suit and pink high heels. "I mean, yoga and meditation help, but I still want what I want when I want it, you know?"

I do. But I don't know how to articulate my thoughts, and I hope someone else in the room might offer some insight. It's a relief not to hear about God all the time. I still flinch a little when I hear the word "God" like I've been caught with my hand in the cookie jar.

"We have to learn to let go of the false self—the ego—completely," says a deeply tanned white man, dressed all in light blue, oozing arrogance. "I've let go of my ego and found great freedom. It's like my Rinpoche always says, as his best student, I must be an example to others." He pauses to let the significance of his words sink in. "You just have to let go. When my yoga teacher asked me to take over teaching his class because I had exceeded his skill level, he told me I had given him the greatest lesson on humility and letting go in his lifetime."

I could barely keep from laughing. Humanity is a mass of contradictions, and it's fun to see people embrace the messiness without apology.

The next woman speaks, and I wonder if she might be Hawaiian. She looks like she just stepped out of a suntan lotion ad, despite her sweatpants and frayed jean shirt. She is so young and fresh-faced; I think maybe she's only here out of curiosity.

"My boyfriend and I were both heroin addicts. He left me one day in Thailand without a word. I didn't have any money or a way home. I was begging in the street when a Buddhist monk asked if I'd like to be free from drugs." She points to the scars on her legs as proof of something but doesn't elaborate. "I knew I couldn't call my mom. My dad had died a few months before, and I didn't even call her, much less go to the funeral. My own dad died, and I just wanted my boyfriend and more and more and more drugs.

"I made a choice and went with the monk to the monastery. There were a lot of other addicts. The monk found me an empty tent and gave me a blanket, a cup, and a plate. They brought us water and some food each day, not much else. They would just sit with us and listen. It was hell, but somehow their devotion to a bunch of messed up kids got to me.

"It was awful and painful and the most amazing experience of my life. It's hard to describe.

"They helped me write a letter to my mom, and that's the only reason I'm home today. She sent me a plane ticket and even wrote she was proud of me. The monks broke my heart open, and my mom stepped in. We are so close now. I can't remember why we used to fight so much. I appreciate all of you being here. It's how I stay clean and that matters to me today more than anything."

I don't feel the tears on my cheeks until a small packet of tissues makes its way around the circle to me. I feel love for everyone in that room. Even the arrogant man, just by being here, is helping her stay clean. When arrogance is humbling, we may be onto something. After the meeting, I sit under a shade tree outside while Samron attends a meditation.

Dear Cave Woman,

There was a lot of talk about the ego at the Buddhist meeting today. How do I make my ego go away?

All this talk about making the ego disappear is nonsensical. The ego is just a lens through which you see yourself and the world. Some people look through the wrong end and see others as tiny and insignificant. Others look at the world through a zoom lens and only focus on one detail. Some go back and forth. You'll gain a more accurate view of yourself with me by your side.

See yourself just as you are, neither diminished nor exaggerated. Without a lens, no picture can form. Without a lens, you can't create a picture of your life. Where would you like to focus your lens?

I'd like to ease my intense focus on the Unreliable Narrator. I'll never get this right. I don't even know who I am.

Focus on me instead, and remember, you're an imperfect human. Be that fully. Rest in the arms of a giant mama gorilla and feel her grooming your hair. Wrap yourself around a festive dolphin and feel pulled through healing saltwater. Restore yourself with a dose of moxie and just sit back for a minute. You can go back to worrying anytime you please.

I promise.

Maybe I should become a Buddhist so I can achieve enlightenment. Can humans really become enlightened?

What modern people call enlightenment is refocusing your lens to see humankind as an ancient animal among many, a small and continuous part of nature.

Humankind has created so many rules focused on perfectionism and shifting the blame instead of living together peacefully. Modern humans don't question what they're told. Learn to question everything, investigate everything, and be willing to learn.

I'll never feel free.

Freedom is learning to throw off the shackles and balance equity with wildness.

What an awful thing to do to ourselves. When did we start to demand unattainable perfection from our clearly imperfect selves?

Humans stumbled—badly—when they attempted to control each other and nature.

We gave ourselves jobs and started fighting over money? We put ourselves to work herding animals?

The agricultural "revolution" and domesticating animals turned humans away from nature.

Did you have livestock?

Why would we do that? Why would we give ourselves and those poor animals full-time jobs? Why would we tether ourselves to the whims of the weather? Why would we want to give up our freedom?

Well, humans did at some point, I'm guessing for a reason.

Humans are inventive. At times, our inventions work against our own nature. Full-time farming and livestock were inventions that turned out poorly for the environment.

More attempts by humans to control the uncontrollable?

You can't harness wildness; instead, you have to move with its inclinations. Before humans tied themselves to jobs, we moved at our own pleasure.

Didn't you say your community lived in one place?

At times we did, but we wandered a great deal. We only did what you would call "work" a few hours a day. The rest of the time, we enjoyed ourselves, shared stories, and created whatever we pleased. When humans domesticated animals and began farming, they domesticated themselves, too. It was also the beginning of overpopulation, pollution, competition, and murder.

Murder? What do you mean?

Humans claimed ownership of the land to raise livestock and to farm. Ownership of the soil had never been an issue before, and it caused problems.

What kinds of problems?

Humans started killing other humans for the first time to claim areas of dirt.

Competition replaced cooperation.

And meat? We started eating a lot of meat?

Meat consumption increased dramatically. Only about ten percent of my communities' diet consisted of meat. It just

wasn't worth the effort when we had an abundance of fruits, nuts, seeds, and vegetables everywhere you looked. Eating as much meat as your people do is just not healthy, for humans, for the animals obviously, or for the planet. With farming, humans also began eating grains, wheat, and sugar in large amounts. Also, not healthy.

What else made us unhealthy?

Living inside and not getting enough sun. Humans need a little sunshine each day for health.

And all this unhealthy craziness led to addiction?

In part, I suppose that's accurate.

I think I'll go to more Buddhist meetings. Different perspectives are helpful.

My new friend joins me under the tree, and I ask, "How was your meditation?"

"Illuminating," she says and adds, "how was your writing?"

"Illuminating," I say, and we smile.

"We can meditate in a lot of different ways. Have you ever been to a tea ceremony? A friend of mine is demonstrating—"

"No, but I'd be very curious," I say.

"Do you have time now?" she asks.

"I sure do," I say and gather up my things, and we go back inside.

Chapter 22

Rage Write

It's been a few weeks since my visit to the emergency room, and I'm well enough to drive short distances. I need the great outdoors. Before Cole left, we'd driven to a reservoir, and I decide to check it out again.

I've taken two weeks off and need to tell them I'm not coming back. I wrote an email explaining why I was quitting and couldn't hit send, so I drove here to vent.

When the reservoir comes into view, the traffic slows. I need to be outside to write about the hurt and anger I still feel. If I'd remained indoors, all this rage might have knocked down some walls. When I'd visited this reservoir in the winter, there hadn't been another car. At seventy degrees, it must have been too cold for native Arizonians.

Today, boats crowd the once-tranquil water. I backtrack a few miles away from prying eyes and park in a gravel pullout. My notebook comes with me as I follow roadrunners up a small canyon. The birds tell me it's okay to rage or to cry but not to put off giving it a voice any longer. I say, "That's why I'm here." They run and bob their heads in agreement.

I put on my small backpack, climb the short distance to a limestone outcropping, sit cross-legged in the dirt, and write.

—◊◊—

Dear Cave Woman,

Maybe I'm hanging around this job waiting for justice. If I don't say something, I think I'll go insane. Help me get some perspective.

I think I can help. Take a minute to look around at the hills and the rocky layers of history that tell stories from millions of lives. Then, imagine a few of those lives.

You're sitting in what used to be the bottom of an ocean. Can you sense the enormity, see the flashes of color, hear the activity, taste the salt, smell the brine?

Some creatures were so unlike anything alive today. Not even the best science fiction could do them justice. Look around and imagine. See them swimming by and getting an eyeful of how bizarre and unexpected you look to them.

I get depressed watching nature shows on TV. They make life seem like an endlessly grim struggle caught in a brutal cycle.

Life is not a grim struggle. Life experiences every possible shape, form, atmosphere, and condition. There is no brutal cycle, only life yielding to transformation without end. Humans obsess over the brutality and miss everything in between.

Humans have lots to recover.

Can you help me transform some of this anger?

Let's start by having you break some sheets of limestone against those jagged rocks. And don't worry. There are no other humans close by.

—⫘—

I get up and easily loosen a piece of limestone from an eight-foot-high outcropping. I lift it above my head, slam down the limestone, and watch as it shatters on the large flat boulders near my feet. The rage cracks and splinters throughout my right arm and shoulder and shatters like a crystal glass. I rub my face and massage my arms until they feel like mine again. I remind myself it's safe to meet this rage with everything I've got.

I think about all the times I didn't listen to my gut. I think about all the people who told me my gut wasn't worth listening to. Damn them all to hell. The rage is fierce, like an electrical fault in a jam-packed fireworks factory, and feels too big to contain in one human body. I rip away more limestone and smash it into the ground. The right side of my face tingles, reminding me of a panic attack. I orient myself back to my body and take a few Spare Tire Breaths. The tingling fades. The first layer of rage lessens. I sit down on the ground. My hands and face are stiff with dirt. The birds are quiet. I notice a small fossil that looks a bit like an elongated shrimp.

—⫘—

Talk to me, Cave Woman.

There are cells in your body from now-extinct creatures. A fossil is not only an imprint left in stone, but ancient graffiti

tagged with the query: Who am I now? That small fossil is an ancestor reminding you how life continues to reshape itself.

And the rage?

The rage is smashing anything that keeps you from forever yielding to transformation.

I'm a human animal on Earth right this second. I'm a woman who has been brainwashed to deny her own power.

And you're reclaiming your power right now. Take a few Volcano Breaths: Do you remember? Breathe in, and as you exhale, constrict your throat just enough that the exhale sounds like the escaping hiss and roar from the mouth of a volcano. Do this several times until you feel stronger. Submerge yourself deep within the planet. Down through the deep layers of laughing mycelium, diving past underground oceans, dense rock, gold, silver, and enormous crystals, to a glowing red room reflecting Earth's core. Hum to send this cleansing vibration up your spine.

Smash another piece of limestone. Smash several more. Enjoy the crackle and thud of rock crashing against rock. Crumble the sandstone between your fingers as the rage clears a path through your body like a plumber's snake through clogged pipes. As you focus on the physical anger, it will change.

Instead of pulling you down, it will lift you up. Where you once felt defeated, you will find determination. Confusion will become clarity.

Feel me by your side, your witness and compatriot. I'm with you, watching, listening, fully immersed in the layers of life, molded by water and wind, all formed by the depth of experience and those that came before.

I do feel determined. The electrical fault has sent the fireworks sky high. Instead of destruction, I now have a power plant. I felt fragile and now feel emboldened. The rage has slowed to a simmer. Rage can be elucidating.

And, one more thing: Damn them all to hell.

Well done. Remember, too, you're also moving some rage your mother couldn't express, that your grandmother wasn't allowed to feel; rage many in your lineage weren't permitted to voice. The rage will come in waves. Let it. As long as you're not hurting anyone, physically expressing your emotions encourages the natural flow of energy throughout your body.

Can you write out the rest of the rage? Can you rage write? I won't look, and you can tear it up.

Oh, yeah, you bet I can rage write.

—⟿—

I stutter step down a steep embankment to a campsite with a metal grate for fires. I write for about ten minutes and then burn my words with a book of matches from our first hotel. I pour water from my water bottle on the ashes and use them to draw a picture of Cave Woman.

I can see the city from here, and it looks tiny like I could crush it with one step. Who knows how much destruction I could cause? I'm still mad, but the rage has subsided. I cry silently and rub the tears, ashes, and dust together on my face.

I'm tired and need to get some rest.

I look up and see a few vultures circling and ask them what they know. They claim to know how to coast through life without expending unnecessary energy. I could learn a thing or two from vultures.

I need sleep. I better head back.

Chapter 23

Good People Exist

It's just barely dawn. The normally dull tan curtains glow slightly orange. This is the first time since I stopped drinking that I didn't wake up when it was still dark. I showered when I got back last night and fell asleep. Miraculous, sanative sleep. I'm delighted and decide to celebrate.

I get a cold bottle of water from the small refrigerator and a towel from the bathroom. I spread the towel across the bed, sit cross-legged, and dump out my backpack contents. It's time for a good cleaning. I wad up and throw away old receipts, notes, and empty wrappers. I collect the change and use a paper towel to wipe down my wallet, notebook, and pens. I fill the sink with warm water in the bathroom, add a few drops of shampoo, and leave my backpack to soak. I find a pen and get back in bed.

Dear Cave Woman,

I experienced strong emotions yesterday and didn't get stuck in a survival response. You've been touting the benefits of feeling emotions. I didn't understand until now. I had a powerful experience of gaining clarity by working with, instead of against, my anger.

You've created safety around feeling emotions, which will—

A question came to me on the drive back yesterday. You helped me expand my view, and I gained a new perspective. How do I see the big picture all the time?

You'll always be jumping between an expanded view and the day-to-day minutia. Just remember to go back and forth between the Long View and the Short View. You need both. Each day write down how you'd like to broaden your perspective and your knowledge, like a wish sent to the womb of the Earth.

My Unreliable Narrator just said, "But people will think I'm a weirdo." So, how do I keep from getting caught up in what other people think? Especially when it hurts? If I quit my job, people will think I did something wrong.

People often believe lies because they can't imagine a good reason for the liar to lie. Give an account from your point of view and stand tall. Most people are defensive and aggressive because they lack knowledge about the Survival Brain. Drop the struggle and simply explain your perspective. You ignored hunch after hunch, which skewed your perspective. You can admit that.

But I've been lied about!

Then speak up and distance yourself from the fallout. If the gaslighting took hold, then you're going to lose this job anyway, so you might as well speak up. Speaking up is very healthy.

I can promise you this: You will feel better speaking up no matter how illogical it seems to your bottom line. Even if nothing observable comes from speaking up, you'll thank yourself later.

I'm afraid to speak up, and I'm scared of the regret I'll feel if I don't speak up.

What matters most? Ask the fear.

—⚏—

I look out the window, let my eyes soften, and ask, "Fear, what helpful message do you have for me?"

—⚏—

Cave Woman?

I'm here. What did fear say?

Fear said, "Keep writing. Eventually, you'll gain clarity, and it will all fade like a dream forgotten upon waking."

Beautiful. Does this situation remind you of anything?

Oh, damn. Yes. My dad and people's misguided adherence to patriarchy. The narrative that If I don't sacrifice myself, I'll be banished. My only worth is what I give away.

Please know there're good people in the world doing good work, people who would never demand you compete with colleagues.

There are colleagues who don't deceive to achieve?

And companies exist that don't turn workplaces into virtual boxing rings.

How would you rather feel about work?

Like I'm a part of something. Like I'm contributing. Expansive and enjoyable. Excited.

That's the antidote. Can you feel it?

I can, but what if I can't maintain that feeling?

You can't, and you don't need to. You eat leafy green vegetables every day (well, almost) but not all day long, right? Have a small serving of expansive joy each day. Like a ritual. Like a prayer.

I'm not sure I can overcome this betrayal at work and all I've lost. I don't want to learn another damn lesson.

Okay, here's the heart of the matter: Your colleagues are very competitive. They're not working there by accident. That comes from the top and will not change.

But it's a self-development company.

And they don't embody the principles they teach for themselves.

It's painful for you because you can feel the inauthenticity. They're losing out by scaring off the sensitive and intuitive, which is their largest potential swath of customers and employees.

Which includes me?

Which includes you. And remember, you rejected how they did business before you understood you were being gaslighted.

Good point. I didn't like the competitiveness. I see. Thank you, that helps.

You're welcome.

But the anxiety is horrible.

How is anxiety here to help?

It said to help me leave the past behind and look forward.

Beautiful.

Chapter 24

New Notebook

I've been on sick leave for two weeks and one day, and I'm not going back. Anger is pushing me to leave the job. Sadness tells me to walk away and to stop looking back. Fear tells me to get out of harm's way. I'm a kaleidoscope of emotions, but I'm feeling and appreciating each one. I feel like I've lived in a city all my life, and I'm just now noticing all the artful details like the chic cobblestones, intricate ironwork, and watchful gargoyles.

I'm incredibly fortunate to have the option to leave and look for a new job.

I've written seven resignation emails. Some longer than others, but I got a lot off my chest. I choose one to send and then sleep on it.

I reread it this morning, checked in with Cave Woman, and hit send.

I'm more energetic than I've been in months.

Fewer people use this pool than the one at the hotel. I sneak a peek and see the pool is empty and put on my bathing suit. By the pool, I kick off my sandals and realize I've forgotten my towel. I retrieve one from my room. I only remember my earplugs as I'm about to jump in the pool. I run back to my room again, laughing. Who cares?

Today swimming feels like flying, and I grin under the water. My legs are strong. Pushing off one side propels me all the way to the other side. I put my arms out to find the edge.

I explained a bit about the gaslighting and gossiping in the email, but I didn't go into much detail. I wrote I'd developed migraines from working long hours on the computer, and I couldn't continue. I don't know who will read it or what stories will be spun about me, and I don't care.

I climb out of the pool, wrap myself inside two large towels, and recline in a lounge chair. I bought a new notebook and open to a fresh page, which I prop against my bent knees.

—◆◆—

Dear Cave Woman,

After this loss, can you tell me which way to go in my life? Will I be successful?

Take a minute and let one thing end before you jump into another. Give yourself some time to grieve what was taken, what was lost. In time, you'll begin to notice what was found. You've already succeeded brilliantly. You didn't use alcohol, and that matters. Just because you left this job doesn't mean your success has gone unnoticed. Your inner hive is elated because you eventually turned to them and heard their contributions. This is true power; listening, hearing, and understanding your brilliant body, inner community, and wise Creative Genius. That affinity will be reflected in your outer world.

I don't feel successful at all.

You found your voice and used it. You eventually got to say no. You've recognized you can exorcise the patterns left by abuse. You learned that patriarchal control, and its vile progeny of sexism, homophobia, racism, and misogyny, can be witnessed in your own life as well as in the wider world. You're not just an observer. You're a participant.

But I—

Don't you see how your confidence has improved? Don't you see how you took back your power from those who had stripped you bare? How what you thought would tear you down has bolstered you up because you finally followed your gut? Your hive thrives on solidarity and the narrative you're rewriting each day. You and Cole are more candid with each other, which makes your relationship better. Can you see you've found some true friends?

But they—

Moments of genuine connectedness will come from seeing your own abilities. It has nothing to do with anyone else. No amount of praise or money can match the healing power of self-regard.

But she—

The person who pushed you out will only know that she can be manipulative and duplicitous. That's not the frequency of success or healing. It's a vicious cycle of merely knowing how to fight or deceive and never feeling truly accomplished.

That reminds me of addiction. Knowing a better way existed but not believing recovery was possible. I wanted proof before I was willing to attempt something so radical, so different. Now I know to begin experimenting when I get that first hunch of something better.

I'll have to go back north. I won't have enough money to stay. I've lost so much.

It may not seem like much with a dwindling bank account, but I promise, it's everything. When the tears have washed away the doubts, the grief has carved a path back to your heart, and the fear has restored your vision, you will have forged a resilient boundary.

Let yourself experience your own tenderness, like the great teacher it is, and then everything from grief to gladness will surge and fade like a searchlight. When you share these feelings with me, you will see kindness and brilliance everywhere you turn. You, my heart flower, have become your own healer.

I put the towels and my notebook on the glass-topped table beside me, lean back, and turn my face to the sun.

Can't Forgive Ourselves

I'm the first to share at a women's meeting today. I tell the room about leaving Maddy and leaving our old lives for a mirage. I tell them how it all finally drove me to get sober. I share about getting screwed over at a job and ending up in the emergency room. I share how I used work the way I once used alcohol. I share how I let myself get used out of habit. I'm nervous but able to talk without my voice shaking too badly.

"I haven't been able to drive lately and asking for rides to meetings and to the grocery store has almost been the hardest part. I sure hate asking for help. But, turns out asking for rides has been amazing because I've gotten to know several of you better. I used to leave meetings as quick as lightning. Now I have to wait for the person driving me home while she talks to people, which forces me to talk to people."

The room laughs, and I do, too. "I'm serious. It took a hell of a lot for me to come out of my shell. Thanks for all the help. And patience." I pause for a moment and then say, "What an amazingly gorgeous, messed-up group of people we are." We laugh again. "I can't believe how different we are and how much we have in common at the same time." I finish my share, and others share about being screwed over and how hard it is to ask for help and release the self-sacrifice habit.

A woman with platinum blonde hair in a flawless ponytail speaks next. "I used to be the person who screwed people over. If we're only as sick as our secrets, then I should be the one in the hospital. I'm not sure how to say this. Give me a second.

"Years ago, before I got sober, I worked for a company that hosted events at local bars and restaurants for corporate retreats. I got the job through my boyfriend, who was also my boss. I wouldn't recommend dating your boss, by the way. Throw in a bunch of alcohol and cocaine, and scruples fly right out the window." She scrunched up her face and groaned.

"Why is this so hard to say? Okay, here goes. Part of my job became scoping out single women and getting them drunk so they'd party with our corporate clients. I was like a pimp, but the women didn't know they were being used. I've felt terrible for years. I wish I could find each of those women and apologize. Unfortunately, we all have things we can't forgive ourselves for, and this is mine. Thanks for listening."

The next woman shares, "I'm Clara. I'm an alcoholic, and the thing I can't forgive myself for is getting my little sister drunk for the first time. I swear, at nineteen, I already knew I was an alcoholic. Both my parents were alcoholics, and I just knew. My sister was sixteen and loved school. She was really good at science and was gonna be an environmentalist. I believe she could have saved the world. I really do. I was so jealous I couldn't stand it. I knew if I talked her into drinking, she might get hooked, too. I hate myself every damn day. I stay away from people because I'm so afraid I'll hurt them. But I have to be here, in these meetings. I have to stay sober. My sister joined a gang in prison. I can hardly believe the hate-filled tattoos she got. She spews hatred, and I'm to blame. I work two jobs and go to meetings. She's in her third rehab, and I'm paying for her to go. I shouldn't admit this, but I'm so damn lonely. I deserve far worse for what I did. The very least I can do is stay in recovery and keep supporting my sister, hoping she'll get here, too."

We talk after the meeting. I ask her what meeting she's going to next, and I ask if she can give me a ride.

"I'll give you a ride. I'm happy to pick you up, but people keep trying to tell me my sister's alcoholism isn't my fault. I don't want to hear it. I'm different from other people. I'm separate from the rest of the world. I deserve to be alone."

"I won't. I promise. I would appreciate a ride, though."

"Can I ask you a question about your sister?" I ask.

"I may not answer it," she says.

"That's fine. One hundred percent your choice. I'm wondering why your sister joined a hate group? It seems like a big leap from a science nerd to joining a hate group."

"I've asked, and she says they're her family. Maybe to punish me for getting her drunk that first time. I think I'm the one she hates, but I'm not sure."

"Thanks for answering," I say, and we make plans for her to give me a ride.

Chapter 25

Hatred, Loneliness, & Innovation

I'm sitting on the closest park bench to my little apartment, wearing a very dark pair of sunglasses. My eyes are still sensitive to the light. The defused light from the setting sun is just bright enough to write by. I can't stop thinking about the woman with the sister in hate groups.

—⚡—

Dear Cave Woman,

Throughout my life, I've had many people confess to me that they feel uniquely alone. Does everyone feel separate?

Many people believe they are uniquely separate and everyone else is happily connected to family and friends. They feel like a lone fish in a sea filled with schools of fish. Do you know what people do when they feel like they don't fit in?

They blame themselves. They think something's wrong with them, and that's why they don't fit in?

That's right. And what do people do when they feel something is wrong with them?

They look for somewhere they do fit in?

Yes, and sometimes they find groups based on a common enemy.

Like the woman in prison who joined hate groups. Why join a group based on hate?

Hate groups manipulate people's emotions and give them someone or something to blame for feeling isolated and empty.

When people have a common enemy, do they feel like they belong?

When people have a common enemy, they become part of a group. They feel like they belong. It's the ultimate irony.

I hate them for hating. I'm prejudiced against prejudiced people. Is that a contradiction?

Hating haters keeps the cycle of hate going.

Love thy enemy?

Not necessarily. When people bond over hatred, they feel justified when their hatred is returned. Your hatred is like fuel for their beliefs.

I don't know how to not hate the haters.

Hatred is an important emotion. Hatred lets you know when your boundaries have been severely trampled, and repair work is in order.

I hate to say this, but hatred does feel good. Like they're bad, and I'm good. Like I'm smart, and they're dumb.

That's precisely what they think.

Well, damn. I hate that!

Hatred is clarifying. There is no ambiguity with hatred. People enjoy feeling certain in their beliefs, but certainty

is unsustainable in an uncertain world. Haters have to keep finding reasons to hate.

Why do we need hatred?

You need hatred to get away from or fight against treacherous situations. But, if you can't get away, hatred will serve as a reminder until you can regain more autonomy and self-determination.

So, what do I do?

Acknowledge your own hatred, even appreciate how powerful and justified you feel. Enjoy the clarity you feel. Write it out.

Then write in detail about what was taken and how it left you vulnerable. What safety net disappeared? Was hope stolen? Was compassion lost? Is there any left? What dreams got buried so you could blend in better?

I don't imagine this can be done in one sitting.

It'll take practice.

What if hatred doesn't resolve?

Practice and persistence are key to any new skill.

Hatred is a skill?

Working with your hatred instead of throwing it at someone is a skill.

I can see why people hold on. I could easily see mistaking hatred for righteousness.

Good insight. People don't understand hatred's message and use it like a shield to conceal their exposed boundaries. They keep looking for reasons to inflame the hatred so they don't feel vulnerable. Unchecked hatred spreads like wildfire.

If you feel hatred and it goes unchecked, you'll obsess over the object of your hatred. Or acting a lot like the people you hate. Either way, there's no resolution.

Do I have to feel empathy for haters?

If you don't understand your own hatred, you'll get caught in a battle with the haters, like two elk with their antlers locked. Writing about your own hatred will energetically disengage you from the tangle of antlers. You'll feel the difference. You'll restore perspective and can then act—or not—from there.

I can neutralize hate?

You'll feel as if you've neutralized hate, but it's just returned to guard duty where it'll be on call if needed, ready to protect.

If I'm feeling emotions all the time, isn't feeling neutral wrong?

Feeling neutral is not wrong. But, I want to emphasize this, it's important; never underestimate the power of feeling neutral.

Aren't I supposed to have high-vibrating emotions, like joy and happiness, all the time to attract good things?

Neutrality is a high-vibrating state. If you measure vibration with hertz, joy is around 550 Hz, love around 500 Hz, guilt around 30 Hz, but neutrality comes in at a nice 250 Hz.

And beating myself up?

Around 20 Hz. You berate yourself for feeling bad, you berate yourself for feeling good, and you even berate yourself for feeling neutral.

Is neutrality different than feeling numb?

Very different. In my life, I felt neutral a lot of the time. Neutrality was a plateau from which to see a reflection of myself and the options that lay before me. I could appraise my life without duress. My Creative Genius and I could appraise my life together.

Neutrality is restorative. A deep sense of neutrality is another thing you missed when you were drinking. You thought alcohol neutralized your thoughts, feelings, aches,

and pains, but it only suppressed them for a time. **Feeling contentedly neutral resets your nervous system. In neutral, I could recognize my Creative Genius with more certainty.**

And get inspired?

Inspiration is the brainchild of neutrality.

Wait a minute. You mean enjoy feeling neutral? Take breaks? Be lazy? No way, kicking back feels like a sin. My dad called me lazybones. I think it was the worst insult he could find. Our culture is horrified by laziness. It's like a mortal sin, rife with judgment.

Let's switch that up. Being lazy is more than okay. Kicking back is vital, especially before or after any new endeavor. A seed can remain a seed long before it begins to grow. Aspects of your life are like seeds in winter, pure potential at rest, getting deep restorative sleep. Some parts are sprouting, testing the soil, the air, and the water, exploring if the conditions and the season align for new growth. Other aspects of your life reach maturity and return to seed once again.

A new life, a new project, a new start all follow a cycle of restoration, exploration, flowering, and returning to seed. If you force a seed to grow outside this natural cycle, it will never blossom.

I've forced ideas so many times. I used the false bravery of alcohol to coerce ideas to sprout. It felt horrible. I've beaten myself up for not being consistently creative, but I was simply ignoring the natural cycle. What a relief. I can rest when I need to rest and let the creativity happen when it happens.

Forcing ideas to sprout before their season gives rise to burnout and chronic exhaustion.

I have to wait until I'm inspired?

Not necessarily. Creativity can be fostered, but it can't be forced. Let your lazybones rest and your wild children out to play. Honoring the natural cycle will give you far less reason

to punish yourself. It's where the magic originates, resting in the current of your Creative Genius.

I needed this. It's beautiful. I feel lighter. I've been punishing myself since I was a child. I'm going to tape a note to my wall that says Lazybones Magic.

What else do humans long for?

Creativity, innovation, camaraderie, to name a few. Relatability is always worth exploring. Anything you can relate to is compelling. Even witnessing a fender bender can bring gladness, not because you derive pleasure from pain, but because you feel connected to a fellow human.

Because we can relate?

Yes, humans long for relatability, which is found in both tragedy and comedy. The shared hilarity of a friend getting her legs tied up in a mess of dog leashes can bring more closeness than hours of conversation. Stumbling is relatable. Vulnerability creates bonds. Vulnerability brings healing, especially with addiction. Relatability is a potent ingredient of a satisfying life.

Racists understand each other. Do they have a satisfying life?

No, because on some level, they know racism is made up. There's only one human race, yet racists pretend otherwise, which takes a lot of energy. They shout louder and feed themselves a steady diet justifying their hatred to keep the truth at bay.

I call Cole and share some of what I've written about in my notebook. He says he can relate, and I laugh. We relate so much I feel I'm falling in love all over again. I feel too happy to sleep, and for the first time, insomnia doesn't bother me at all.

Jonesing

Dear Cave Woman,

I want to go back to work even if I end up in the ER again. I'm seriously jonesing for work. The anxiety is overwhelming. I need to drown out this anxiety.

Since anxiety helps you focus on completing your to-do list, drowning it out is impossible. You always have a to-do list running through your mind.

Are you seriously going to tell me anxiety is helpful?

Without a doubt, but remember I'm not talking about a survival response or panic or terror. Anxiety gets you moving. Anxiety motivates you to work on what needs to be completed.

I've always wanted a business card that said, "I get shit done."

You get a lot done because anxiety helps you finish projects.

But I push past the signals from my body when I need a break?

Yes, but now you're learning to recognize the Yellow Caution Zone and taking stock. Yes?

Yes, I am. Why am I having so much anxiety now?

Because recovery is an ongoing project, and anxiety is helping you stay on course.

If recovery is a lifelong project, will I have anxiety forever? If so, I'll start drinking right now.

Addiction makes anxiety worse because working obsessively or drinking is never your true heart's desire. Anxiety may be an aggravating taskmaster but work with it, and you'll—

You make it sound so easy. Anxiety feels awful. How can I bear these feelings?

You can bear those feelings because you are bearing them. When you know that anxiety is cheering you on, you'll develop a different relationship. Anxiety will help you focus and not run into the weeds trying to complete a dozen different projects simultaneously.

I have a long to-do list. My list started at a young age with things like fighting for women's rights, eliminate prejudice, work toward social justice, make musical instruments, sit up straighter, turn everyone into an animal lover, become an anthropologist and a social scientist, learn Spanish, alphabetize my spice rack, make my own lotions and potions, swim every day, build a house—

And I know you could go on and on. You're carrying around a long to-do list. Let's pare it down so anxiety isn't urging you to complete things that aren't realistic or desirable anymore. Teach your anxiety that while you did—for a day—want to learn to build musical instruments, you can safely take that off the list. Is that right?

Yes, I agree.

List all the things you've ever hoped to accomplish and strike off what can go. Then list all the things you've accomplished. Your anxiety needs to know what can be moved from the to-do list to the already done list.

Cole and I built a bunch of tiny houses.

Do you want to build another house?

I guess I still have those on my to-do list. I was hoping we'd build another house someday, but I think I've accomplished enough in that department.

Can you see how lying in bed with "build a house" on your to-do list might add to the pressure you feel?

Oh, crap. No wonder I feel so much anxiety. Can I keep some hopes for the future without increasing the anxiety?

Absolutely. Prioritize your list. What matters to you at *this moment?*

Stay in recovery is number one?

Naturally. For larger societal goals, write one thing you can do today.

Call another woman in recovery?

Exactly like that.

What if the anxiety still doesn't ease up?

Use your anger to remind anxiety that you're on the case and it can step back.

Does that work?

Of course. Anxiety needs reminders, too.

—⁓—

Radical Act

I call Danny, the woman I met who was having a hard time with her boss. She'd sent me her resume, and I spruced up the design and sent it back. Not only has she found a new job, but now she's the boss and dedicated to treating her employees like she's always wanted to be treated. She sounds happy. I fill her in on what's been happening with me. She offers me a ride to a meeting, and I accept.

After the meeting, I feel tired but guilty for sitting around so much. I do some sit-ups on the floor but feel worn out after only eight. Now I feel tired, silly, and guilty. It might be best just to find my pen and notebook.

—⁓—

Dear Cave Woman,

I heard a saying during the meeting this evening: "Move a muscle, change a thought." Everyone was talking about the necessity of taking action. Do I need to take action? How do I take action when I don't want to move and feel wholly depleted?

When your Unreliable Narrator verbally berates you, it zaps your energy. It's common in your world to use self-flagellation to push yourself, but worry and dread are poor substitutes for inspiration and moxie.

I don't feel inspired at all.

How could you with a condescending commentary dogging your every step?

When you put it that way, I can see the absurdity of thrashing myself into inspiration.

Your Unreliable Narrator tells you it's dangerous not to stay busy all the time.

Busyness has become a habit used for distraction.

Not another habit!

Needing a constant distraction is a core habit. One that gives rise to other habits.

I realize I need to look at things differently.

That's what we do together. In a world motivated by worry and perfectionism, choosing to rescript the Unreliable Narrator is a radical act.

As you rewrite distressing scripts and replace them with supportive words, your nervous system will be less tense. You'll notice the difference in all areas of your life.

No more tension?

You'll never be tension-free because the body needs some tension to function.

Tension is natural. Chronic pressure is not. Don't expect complete freedom from tension.

And then I take action?

No. Then you take a nap. You're tired and can barely move. Rest always comes first. Actually, rest comes first, in the middle, once again, routinely, over and over again, and again in the end.

Because rest is when the magic happens?

Without a doubt. Indubitably. Unquestionably.

Okay, okay. What are you, Ms. Thesaurus, today?

Add in some curiosity, and you can make magic at will. Lazybones magic.

Chapter 26

Impossible to Duplicate

I sit down in a folding metal chair before a meeting and hug my backpack for comfort.

A woman next to me says, "I've been watching you," and scans me from foot to nose. Then she says, "You interest me."

Uh-oh, I think. I recognize that tone and I don't want to be someone's project. Before I can say I don't care if I interest her or not, she says, "You should sit up straighter. Get a real purse. You're a grown woman, not a kid who needs a backpack for school supplies."

I put up my hand and say, "This isn't *My Fair Lady*, and I'm not a flower girl in need of diction lessons. I'll decide what changes, if any, I want to make." I stand up to move to another seat. As I walk away, she says, "And get some clothes that fit. I can't even make out your figure in those baggy clothes."

Good, I think, my body is none of her business.

Even though I moved away from her, I feel distorted. My cheeks feel enormous, like chipmunk cheeks filled with sunflower seeds. My legs pull away from me, bizarrely long, like pulled taffy. My torso folds like a deflated accordion with a hunchback, squat and distended. I feel everyone's eyes on me, unable to turn away from the hideous monster I truly am. No wonder Cole left. I'm the Creature from the Black Lagoon, and Cole was too nice to say anything. He'll never want me back.

I'm irritated and leave the meeting. I call Odell and tell her why I got irritated enough to leave a meeting early. She reminds me I'm supposed to be resting, so I head back to my place. She also asks how I let the comments from one busybody make me feel so rotten.

On the drive home, I notice how the Unreliable Narrator instantly echoed the insults from the busybody. I put things right by sifting through the fear, the hurt, the self-recrimination, and then breathing my way back into my body, waiting to settle.

Once I'm home, Cole calls for no reason, the most heart-warming reason of all. He's awaiting the delivery of a bronze sculpture at a home he caretakes. He'd looked at a few apartments but said he could hear the neighbors through the walls or walking above. If one looked or sounded promising, I asked him to send me pictures. We agreed to talk later, and I go outside with my notebook and sit in the chair on my little cement porch. The clouds provide cover for my still-sensitive eyes.

—w—

Dear Cave Woman,

How do I screen out dangerous people?

You just did at the meeting today. You'll feel it in your gut when you meet someone dangerous. Early in your life, sankes conditioned you to override your initial gut reactions. Even though you were taught not to speak up, your body knows.

You'll learn to pick up on the subtler clues. You'll become an ace detective. For now, observe the reaction in your body and check your impressions with those you already know are trustworthy.

Yeah, I did, didn't I? And I recognized how the Unreliable Narrator promptly iterated her words. I think I'd feel better about it if my bladder didn't hurt so much right now. I'm worried about the pain.

Everything you've been doing to stay in recovery will ease your pelvic pain and give your nervous system far more flexibility and resilience.

Can we go over everything again to address the pain?

Yes, when you get settled. What a good idea.

I feel sorry for my nervous system if it's relying on me for comfort. How did you move pent-up crazy-making energy?

We danced, chanted, sang, keened, cried, cleaved, kvetched, groaned, shook, and shouted until we fell to the ground in relief or agony or laughter and then we sang and danced again. We also threw tantrums. Tantrums are a wonderful release at any age. Hit the floor and kick your arms and legs. Holler, moan, or bellow. Do what you need to do to keep those emotions in motion.

If I throw a tantrum, my body will be less tight, and my mind will relax?

Your body is your best friend and can help relieve your overburdened mind. When you intentionally disperse tension by crying, talking, singing, daydreaming, humming, writing, stretching, swimming—and a million other non-addictive ways—your body will release relaxing hormones that help restore a sense of wellbeing.

The ways I've treated my body are awful. I drank and smoked. I ate junk food in a futile attempt to soak up all the poison. I hated my poor body because that's what I was taught.

Like a faithful dog, your body forgives the past.

"Please forgive me, body." Nope, didn't help. I'm ashamed to say I still hate my body.

Nature has provided a physical miracle. Modern people are taught to hate their bodies and judge other people's bodies. This is such an absurd thing. Your body is a profound accumulation of trillions of cells and millions of years, a recipe impossible to duplicate.

But it's—

Your body is your greatest collaborator and finest confidant.

You and your body are literally soul mates.

We judge our bodies, and the self-hate causes us to judge how others look? That's tragic. Now I'm crying.

It's so good to cry. You'll have more room for input from your Creative Genius.

Yay, right. I've heard that before. I'm a spiritual being having a physical experience.

Or something like that.

You're an energetic being, being particularly energetic at this precise moment. All energy gets recycled, morphs, transforms, and changes. There is life you can see and touch, and life you cannot see or touch, but it's all life.

A cell in your body may once have been a cell in an octopus ten million years ago. That tiny octopi cell is part of you. There is information communicated to you through that octopi cell that informs your point of view. If you tune in, you can find out about life and how to live it, about death and how to die, and everything in between.

I always knew I wasn't entirely human.

My community knew that our bodies were once part of other animals and other things. We used that to our advantage. Our fastest runner had cheetah energy. Our best tree climber had lizard energy.

We're literally made from the past?

Your body is a reunion of energy pulled together, making one beautiful and unique human. Together and without self-hate, you'll get to see beyond the mystery that judgment has stolen.

I feel like an ingrate. And terribly guilty.

This is guilt from the past that you can quit.

Just like that?

Yes, just like that.

Okay, but now I'm bored. How can I be so consumed with trauma and drama and then simply feel bored?

Boredom is anger that's gone stale, a sign you may need to use your physical self to release stagnated anger. Let the anger propel you out of lethargy enough to sing, dance, talk, pick up the phone, or say hello to a neighbor on the way to the laundry room. Better yet, ask your body what it would like. Your body knows how to mend and renew itself. Your body craves interaction.

When you meet your body on this level, systems come into balance, wisdom intervenes, and trauma transforms.

Let me tell you a story.

I went below ground with the other women to tell our stories on the cave walls. As I made my way from one cave to another, I slid down a narrow, smooth tube. I lost my bearing and slipped into a crevice. My arm jammed, and my head lodged in what felt like a mouth full of jagged teeth. After a slight bit of maneuvering, I could tell I was stuck. Panic filled my body, and I screamed and fought until I bled. I thought no one could hear me. Dread filled my body, and I stopped moving and screaming, and I couldn't even speak. The freeze response helped numb the pain as I felt my life slip away. I knew what was happening because I'd been taught by my elders this can occur when we're caught by a predator. We freeze when we can't run away or fighting against a predator hasn't worked. As animals, we don't choose the freeze response. Our survival system does. I felt like there was a terrified cheetah running around my stomach, but I could no longer speak or move. I felt fear so acutely that I wished death would come quickly.

I could hear voices far away. They spoke for what seemed like a long time. Then I heard very soft singing. Songs I knew well. One woman walked toward me so quietly I didn't hear her footsteps. I only heard her voice get slightly louder than the rest of the voices. She would stop moving, then move forward again. She spoke to my statue-like body and asked to be guided. She delicately put her hand on my foot and kneaded it with tenderness. She tenderly moved her hands up my legs, which called me back into my body. She reassured me again and again that we are amazing, life is amazing, and amazing things were still to come. She rested her hand on my low back and sang about resilience and strength.

She placed her hand over my heart and merged it with her own. I could feel her tenderness. I could feel her heartbeat. I was able to breathe, and tears clouded my vision.

My free arm began to shake, and she reassured me that was the key to getting free. After the shaking subsided, I felt her hands deftly reach between the rock and my body, surround my stuck arm, and slowly pull it free. With a reach that seemed impossible to me, her hands wrapped my head and freed it from the jaw of jagged rocks. After I was free, the women sat in a circle around me. Not too close yet close enough to hand me a flask filled with water. I felt exposed and vulnerable. I couldn't meet their eyes. They asked me to lay on the sand floor and assume the same awkward position I had contorted into in the crevice. Then they asked me to practice coming out of the position several times to give my body the felt sense that the difficulty had passed. I did the best I could. Then I kicked and writhed like a snake and roared like a wild cat. I felt such rage. I understood wanting to kill. As I felt the rage, it morphed into a spear of grief that ran through me and ushered out a flood of tears. I rocked back and forth, and the women joined my rhythmic movement and raspy vocalizations, each expressing their own grief, fear, anger, or elation. Finally, I smiled, and we laughed together. I could look each woman in the eye. My ordeal was over. I was alive and back with my wise and loving community.

I remember the experience vividly, but I've never had to relive it. I've never had a flashback or been retraumatized by the memory. I happily returned to the cave many times in my life.

Did you know women painted much of the art found in ancient caves? Who else would bring our world to life in the womb of the Earth?

Family Dining

I slept fairly well last night, considering I'm meeting family for dinner tonight. Usually, nerves would keep me awake, wondering how my dad would remind everyone I'm to blame for all bad things. Cole and I talk several times during the day. On the third call, he asks what I'd think of buying the company where he currently works.

"Cold," I answer.

"That's true, but we'd be together," he says.

"We'd keep each other warm?" I ask.

"Think about it and let me know?"

"I will. I love you loads, and I'm not sure buying a company you don't even like working for is a loving thing to do."

"True, but it would be ours."

"Okay, I'll give it some thought," I say, and we promise to talk after dinner.

My father, a retired government lawyer, my brother, a practicing lawyer, and my nephew, a soon-to-be lawyer, are in Phoenix because my brother is attending a law conference and asked Dad and his son to come along to play golf. They have time to meet for one dinner, and I don't feel like I can say no. I'm nervous, and I've arranged to check in with a few sober friends after dinner. I also have a meeting list if I need some extra support later tonight.

I drive to the restaurant, park, and wait in my car. As they enter the restaurant through a tall glass door, I catch up as the hostess asks how many for dinner.

We hug lightly and without much enthusiasm. We're not close, and they all know I wasn't a fan of how my dad abused my mom. I doubt my nephew knows anything other than his grandma passed

away from Alzheimer's. I'm not here to argue. I hope to avoid arguing, which seems an absurd goal for any endeavor.

We sit, and the hostess hands us menus. We smile at her broader
than we do with each other.

Tall sparkling windows face the parking lot in a large semi-circle. The
massive tieback curtains and carpet with large strokes of red and orange
dampen the sound. I wonder how they keep the carpet looking so clean.

My dad orders a glass of wine. My nephew and brother are
non-drinkers and say water is fine. Water is fine for me too, I say. I
never did drink much around my family, so no one comments.

We make chit-chat about golf, which I don't play or watch or
care a thing about. I tell them I just finished a freelance job and I'm
leaving in a few weeks.

I wait for my dad to start reinforcing his story about me. My brother
is his biggest supporter and believes I'm the bad seed. They all do. Being
with them only makes me miss my mom more. Despite decades of propaganda, my mom never bought into the bad seed version of me. That
must have driven my dad nuts. I'm glad the food arrives quickly.

I enjoy two mouthfuls of creamy pasta before he begins. It's payback time for saying anything about him abusing my mom.

"So Haiti didn't work out. I had a feeling you were chasing rainbows."

I was wrong. He was right. Point to Dad. "Nope, but at least we
tried. Nothing ventured, nothing gained, right?" I try.

No response. Everyone looks at their plate.

"It's typical. Par for the course," my dad says. "But I think what
matters now is getting a handle on your life. I know you have these"—
he shakes his bony hands near his chest like he's being electrocut-
ed—"feelings. But it's time to get over this hyper sentimentality. It's
not good for you."

I stare and wait for him to continue because there's no answer for
being bad because I have feelings.

But my nephew and brother nod yes, so I guess I'm wrong. He's right. I sink a bit in my chair.

My nephew chimes in and says, "Grandpa has done so much for me. I'm sure you feel the same." He smiles and gestures his water glass to his beloved grandpa. My brother meets my eye and nods yes. I guess I'm supposed to congratulate my dad, so I do.

"Yes, so much," I say.

Dad looks down and smiles with pride. He looks satisfied. Praise makes him happy.

"I know we don't talk much. Answer your phone once in a while, why don't you?"

I open my mouth to answer.

Maybe I look hurt because he quickly adds, "I'm just kidding."

They laugh. I don't hear the joke, but I fake smile and say, "I really could answer my phone more. That's true." I'm not lying. I didn't answer my phone much when obsessing over work.

I slump further in my chair.

"If I made some mistakes in my long life, I'm sorry," Dad offers with a frowny face.

My brother lowers his voice to add authority and says, "You should accept his apology."

Somehow, I've been given the power to forgive someone's whole life. Why not, I think. I didn't know bad seeds could grant absolution. Tears threaten, and I twist my face to keep them inside because once again, I'm at fault if I don't forgive.

"Oh, here we go. Here come the waterworks. Don't get hysterical," Dad says.

"I'm not hysterical. I'm just so happy to see you all," I lie and lay it on thick. Truly, why not? "And, I'll add," I say, "if I made any mistakes in my long life, I'm sorry, too."

"Finally," Dad says. "I've waited all my life to hear that."

Everyone smiles but me.

I'm confused, but that's always been the point. Confuse Sil and make Dad look good no matter what. But what I don't say is this: They can have their "bad seed" story, they can get me to lie to avoid confrontation, but they absolutely cannot have my sobriety. I feel such a flood of relief. I promise my hive a good cry for the ride home.

"Here's the thing we wanted to ask you," says my brother.

Now that my head is spinning, and I can't think straight, here comes the ask.

"Dad would like to buy a condo here, and amazingly he'd like you to share it with him. Isn't that great?"

"Amazing," my nephew echoes.

"You mean take care of Dad?" I ask.

"We'll no, but you'd be expected to help out with meals and cleaning and running errands."

"That pretty much sounds like taking care of Dad," I repeat.

My brother chuckles and says, "But Dad would be doing you a big favor, and you'd help out in return."

I remember one time I got really brave and asked my dad straight up, "Why are you so mean to me?"

For a brief moment, he stepped away from his role and said, "So you'll have to take care of me when I'm old." And here we are. The youngest daughter, like a seventeenth-century novel, expected to serve the aging patriarch.

If my recovery was not shining inside me like a diamond, clearing my mind of all the gaslighting, I might have said yes. I love this city, and the imposed confusion might have led me to capitulate.

I excuse myself and go to the bathroom. I lean over the sink and start laughing. I must sound crazy because a woman exits a stall and asks if I'm okay. I stop laughing and smile. "Yes, just crazy family stuff." I wave my hands like I'm trying hard not to laugh more.

"Oh, I understand family craziness. I'm glad you can laugh."

"I am too." I shake my head, grinning. "I'd explain but I wouldn't even know where to begin."

"I'd start at the end where you're able to laugh," she says.

"Excellent point. Thank you." Time to put this terrible idea of an evening to bed.

As I walk back to the table, I know I want to own a company. Cole is my family and I'd like to have a family business. I walk tall and feel a tiny thrill near my heart.

I return to my seat and tell them I'm returning north. I announce Cole and I are buying the business where he works.

They look offended and tell me I'm not grateful. That it won't work out. I'll fail like I did with my "Haiti foolishness" as my dad calls our canceled trip. But they're wrong, and all points go to recovery.

I thank them for dinner and say I need to get going. I offer to chip in, but they tell me they'll pay. I thank them again and make my way across the colorful carpet. I'm surprised it's still light out. Feels like I've been here for hours. After driving a few blocks, I pull into the parking lot of a tire store and call Odell before heading home. I feel sad. Somehow knew I would. Sadness feels right. I cry as I drive home.

In my tiny kitchen, I brew a cup of chamomile tea in the microwave and gingerly take it with me to bed. I bought a new pack of colored pens. Where did I put those?

—⋙—

Dear Cave Woman,

You talk a lot about becoming a whole human again. I'm missing a big piece of myself. My mom's gone, and she was my champion. I miss her fiercely, and I feel sorry for myself. Will I ever feel whole without her?

You might be surprised by what you discover as you regain wholeness.

I'll get my mom back?

In a sense, yes.

But I'll still feel stuff?

Of course. "Feeling stuff" also includes missing your mom, loving your mom, and sharing your sadness and memories. Also talking to her, hearing her voice again.

Then I definitely want to be whole. What parts of my inner hive got cocooned and why? Can you give me examples?

The parts of yourself that drew attention during dangerous times: That little girl who spoke her mind and didn't understand why that caused trouble. That angry teenager who lit fires and beat drums and drew the attention of people with ill intent.

I want these parts back. I need my full crew, my full voice. I can guess more of the aspects that were cocooned. The one who spoke her mind. The one who was teased for feeling wonder. The one who got teased for not being attractive enough. The one who got dangerous attention for being attractive.

The Survival Brain quieted these aspects of yourself, which was lifesaving and meant to be temporary.

If they were quieted for my protection, why didn't they return when I needed them again?

You didn't know they were missing or in need of retrieval. You didn't know how to call them home.

How do I invite them back? Do I send a bee-vite?

First, get tactile. Rub your hands together, touch your shoulders or the front of your thighs as touchpoints to bring you more fully into your physical self.

I've listened to so many meditations where they tell you to ignore the body like it's a spare part you can stuff in a drawer.

Being present in your body helps call them home.

Okay, I can feel my body. Oh, wow, I can feel my knees. They each feel like a whirlpool gently circulating. What's next?

Imagine the hive of your heart filled with bees making their own nourishing elixir. Notice some cells are empty. What aspects of yourself were quieted when danger lurked? Right now, what do you feel is missing?

I feel a lack of enthusiasm for starting over again.

Good insight. Do you remember when or where you lost some of your enthusiasm?

Well, yeah. School. There is probably a very enthusiastic bee at each school I ever attended.

Now, invite those enthusiastic bees home.

Imagine the bees traveling at the speed of light back to your hive. Picture them crawling through the entrance and arriving to a wave of raucous cheers. Feel the joy of all the other bees who have been working away without much enthusiasm. Feel the relief and joy. Feel the buzz.

My whole body is buzzing. I feel clearer, more fiery. But I still don't feel much enthusiasm for returning north.

Enthusiasm is on board but will need some time to acclimatize. Let enthusiasm percolate at its own pace. What else do you feel is lacking?

I don't have much presence. Is presence something you're born with, or did I lose my Earth-goddess presence somewhere along the way?

Oh, your Earth-goddess presence was suppressed and stripped away. Do you recall times when your presence was depleted?

I can't recall a specific time, but I can feel the sensation of shrinking and fading into almost nothing each time I was dismissed.

Claim your presence with lionhearted ferocity. Don't be shy. Bring your wrath to stand for any unjust banishment. Cry and march and chant and stomp to reclaim yourself. Throw a tantrum, if need be. Or dance.

—⚏—

I feel desperate enough to lay on the floor and kick my legs and arms in the air. After a minute, I get into it and curse and punch and rock side to side and back and forth along my spine. I say aloud, "Help me be whole again," and hope no one can hear me.

I cry, which is quite painful, but it feels like healing pain instead of inflicted pain. I persist and let myself feel my body feeling the healing pain.

—⚏—

Dear Cave Woman,

I don't feel like writing anymore. I'm ashamed to say I just want to wallow in self-pity for a while.

That's awesome.

How on Earth is self-pity awesome?

First, let me commend you for throwing a tantrum to bring scattered aspects of your hive back home. You were vulnerable to abuse without these aspects. You are safer now, a powerhouse of wholeness.

Self-pity helps me? That's craziness. Although, I'll admit self-pity does feel kinda cozy.

Self-pity calls you into its arms like a soft blanket and invites tears to flow. Self-pity helps you lean into grief.

But I beat myself up like crazy for feeling sorry for myself. I left my cat. It was the worst thing I could have done, but so many people have it much worse. How dare I feel sorry for myself.

How dare you not feel sorry for yourself. Without the self-pity and the sadness it brings, you wouldn't be able to grieve. Without grieving, wounds stay in the dark and grow, like mold, creating mental and physical distress, not to mention the consequences it creates for those around you. Grieving is necessary healing work. Unresolved grief leads to great tragedies.

What if I fall into self-pity and can never get out? Then what?

If self-pity becomes unrelenting, you'll seek to distract yourself. Pay attention when you crave unhealthy diversions. You'll usually find you're avoiding an emotion. Noticing is powerful and helpful. Conferring with emotions is the *pièce de résistance*.

All these emotions to manage. I'll never gain any stupid wisdom. The self-pity, pain, grief, regret, shame, blame, rage…oh, my gosh, the list is endless!

It feels endless because pushing emotions away is more familiar. Take heart.

You're learning to garner the energy they bring.

And you're right, you may never be wise, but you will be wiser.

Wanting to wallow in self-pity is sage advice from your Creative Genius.

How can I tell the difference between the sage advice and all the other craziness inside my brain?

You just answered your own question. One feels like sage advice, and the other feels like craziness.

Let me tell you a story.

A lone man circled our tribe for a few weeks. Being alone was very unusual, so we watched him closely. We could feel him alternating between rage and worry. We didn't know if he would approach peacefully or aggressively or just attempt to take some food. We didn't venture outside our community and did our best to conduct our usual activities to demonstrate we weren't in distress and had plenty to share. We wanted to send the signal that he could approach and that we would listen to his story.

He finally stepped out from behind a tree a great distance away to let himself be seen. He did that for a short time, each day, for three days, before we sent a group of diplomats to meet him. They approached him slowly, a few steps at a time, so as not to frighten him away.

The diplomats returned to the village with the frightened lone wolf who tried to appear nonchalant. He concealed his emotions, indicating his understandable suspicion. We concealed very little from each other. Hiding our feelings or intuitive hits could have obscured a problem that might have threatened the entire community. If one of us had a premonition about a predator or natural disaster and chose to ignore that feeling, it could imperil us all.

He continued to protect himself by telling us several versions of what had happened. We listened for the true story behind his words. One story he told was that he'd been separated while hunting. He said his fellow hunters left while he was sleeping, which made no sense to us. He also told us he was kidnapped during an attack and then escaped. Because of these varied stories, we knew whatever had happened left him so traumatized even talking about it felt dangerous. We could tell at this point he was not a threat to us and that the community of his birth had somehow all perished. We did not push him to do or say anything. Our first task was to convince him we were safe, so we went about our daily lives and let him receive the comfort of our routine. Witnessing us go about our business would be bittersweet for him. A reminder of all he had lost. But he needed to experience for himself that he was welcome, that he was safe with us if he decided to stay.

Cave Woman?

Yes?

Did he stay? Did you think he was crazy?

Your people would call this person crazy. We knew the enormity of his loss, and we knew he was having an appropriate reaction. He worked hard to fight the grief as long as possible. The so-called "craziness" reflected the hopelessness from losing his original community. We understood, and we knew any of us could suffer such a loss.

What happened? Was he okay?

Slowly, we gave him food, water, and reasons to trust us, reminding him in simple ways and with great patience why he was extraordinary and why and how he belonged.

He lost his community; that was the initial trauma. The same trauma reverberates throughout humanity today.

Addiction started with the loss of healthy communities. A loss everyone can sense.

I worry feeling lost will swallow us whole. I hope we can find a way to get filled up without abuse or addictions. I worry we rage or wallow in fear as a way to fill ourselves up.

Loss doesn't keep you from longing. Blame doesn't prevent shame. You can't constantly beat yourself up and find self-regard.

What happened to your lone wolf?

We saw the rage in our lone wolf. At first, he paced with balled fists, talking to himself. His grief surfaced, and he fought to keep it at bay. He would sink to the ground and cry and then threaten anyone who came near him. His eyes darted from side to side, and he would grab pots and jars and smash them on the ground. He struggled so viciously, and at times we feared his rage and grief might smother our lone wolf. He would groan and hold his head to keep the truth of his loss from being known.

Did you ever find out what happened to him?

His story did emerge eventually. He was the only one to survive a natural disaster, which left him grieving an incalculable loss alone.

Did he accept your community as his? Did he ever feel at home?

Eventually, our lone wolf let us care for him, and we let him care for us. We loved him. For a time, our lives became an extended grief ritual.

No matter how we might rage or grieve, we catch each other. We are catching you now.

—〰—

I call Cole, wake him up, but he's glad I called. I tell him I want us to buy the company. I want a place of our own, too. But I must ask, "Are you sure you want me to come back?"

"I'm sure," he says simply.

"How do you know you're sure?" I press.

"Because I always wanted you to come home, but I needed you to decide on your own," Cole says.

"What more could I ask for?" I ask.

"What more could you possibly need?" Cole quips.

I laugh and say, "You know, you're right. All I ever needed was for you to love me while I recovered. I think that's all anyone in recovery needs. I'm very lucky."

"I'd say we're both lucky."

Loved Anyway

I'm amazed I have girlfriends. I've told them almost everything, and they're still my friends. Not only do they know my darkest, most shameful secrets, but they want to throw me a party. I'm floored. They've seen me cry. They know the things I'll never forgive myself for, and yet they said I should pick the restaurant for my going away party. There are some rotten people in the world, but I'm starting to wonder if the good might just outweigh the bad.

I picked a vegan restaurant after Marian said it was her favorite place to eat. The dining room is narrow and tall with exposed ductwork, and the air smells like cinnamon and chiles. Paintings of desert plants line the bright white walls. After everyone arrives, we order at the counter in the back. They'll bring our food to the table. We push three tables together. Pineapple tops sit in mason jars with roots dangling in the water and serve as centerpieces. The restaurant is bustling, but not so loud we can't hear each other.

Our food arrives before any awkward silences. I ordered the lasagna, and it's so amazing I refuse to share a single bit.

"Sylvia, be nice and share," commands Odell.

"No f-ing way," I proclaim with a mouthful of the best lasagna I've ever tasted.

Odell reaches her fork toward my plate, and I quickly move my plate out of her reach. I laugh and say, "You all get to come here again. I need to savor every bite."

Laila takes charge and orders more lasagna so everyone can share.

As three plates of lasagna make their way around the table of nine women, we declare it the best dish ever.

Jane takes a bite and states quite seriously, "I don't blame Sil for wanting this all to herself. In fact, I'm keeping this one. Sorry. I can't help it." We watch as she takes another bite, then give her a rousing round of applause.

Jane is known for her utter selflessness, and this is a major achievement.

Wrapped packages make their way from hand to hand and are placed in front of me. A lump forms in my throat, and I have to drink water to swallow.

"I didn't expect this. But, damn, I deserve all the gifts."

Thank goodness everyone laughs. I feel seen and heard and loved anyway. What could be better?

Each package was wrapped with care. "I've never understood when people said the wrapping is so pretty, they don't want to tear it." My voice wavers while I say, "Until now," and add, "I really don't deserve all this."

Odell says insightfully, "You know all our mistakes and love us anyway. Let us return the favor."

"But," I say, "you're all so wonderful. I'd forgive any of you anything."

"That's how we feel about you," says Charlotte.

"Okay, okay, okay…." I stammer. "Me, really? I'm mean, okay, thank you." I sit up straighter, bow my head, and grin as I hear Cave Woman urging me to enjoy the moment.

I receive several recovery books, and Rosa knitted me a hand-made scarf in rich fall colors from amber to apricot.

"I love it," I say. "You made this? It's gorgeous."

"Oh, please," says Rosa. "I love to knit, but who am I going to knit for in the desert? You did me a favor, my dear. In fact, let me know if you want more."

"I'll treasure it. I'll treasure each of you. You all have a piece of my heart. Forever." I look down, wondering if I'll cry, but I don't. I feel good. Really good. I do a little dance in my seat and shimmy my hips and head.

"There's one more," says Marian, who owns a health food store and the one who suggested this delicious restaurant.

I was avoiding this one because it looks like a six-pack wrapped in brown paper tied with raffia. Turns out I was right. But it's a six-pack of various vegetable juices.

Marian says, "We all have some catching up to do in the nutrient department." She lifts her water glass and adds, "To your good health." Everyone raises her glass and says, "To good health."

Odell adds, "To recovery. I mean it. You better stay sober."

"I'll call you every day. How's that?" I ask, grinning.

"I'd like that. I'd like that very much."

Receptive & Sheltered

I arrange my presents across the coffee table back at my place like a kid with a haul of birthday gifts. I delight in them without a hint of shame. Despite playing with my presents like a kid, I get that mellow feeling again of being a grown-up. I thought feeling like an adult would be confining, but I feel freer than ever, like a cave near the ocean, sheltered but with deep water splashing around inside.

A flutter of worry about leaving Phoenix surfaces, and I decide to check in with Cave Woman before I clutter this good feeling with my habitual pessimism.

—⁂—

Dear Cave Woman,

When I get back to the north, how will I know if I've found a healthy community?

You'll need to mix and match. Find a bit here and a bit there. Please be wary of any recovery group that excludes anyone. Look for support groups that understand trauma and post-traumatic stress.

I guess I need to accept that we're social animals.

We would not have multiplied and spread across the globe so rapidly if we weren't social animals.

We need to learn to communicate better.

Ironically, human beings developed extensive communication skills because we survived by working together.

And now we use communication to hurt each other. We may need each other, but we sure don't need people who aim to tear us down.

Modern people need to rise up against those causing harm.

How do I know who to trust?

You're learning to read the energy of the world around you. Learning who to trust takes practice and honing your High Perceiver skills.

I've read about this, and I don't want it. I'm an empath, right? I've read I can't even go to the grocery store without being bombarded by everyone's energy. I feel like a professional victim.

Yes, you are highly perceptive, which was a valued skill in my community. And, no, you're not a professional victim anymore. Do you dread going to the grocery store?

Not really. I kind of like grocery shopping.

That's right. And do you generally need to recover once you've been around people?

Yes, I think so. But I actually like spending time alone.

There's a big difference between needing time alone and enjoying time alone.

When you go out, do you feel like you've absorbed doom and gloom and anguish?

No, that only happens when I see or read about the awful things humans do to other humans. Or when I'm dealing with a sanke.

That's right. See why it's so important to question what you hear? You've been told you're fated to be a victim simply because you can sense and interpret energy. But you're an energy detective. You pick up on information about people and events, and you think it makes you vulnerable instead of more powerful. You've shut yourself down because you've read that if you embrace your High Perceiver skills, you'll be filled with negativity and be abused by sankes.

Yes, I'm very vulnerable, and I attract sankes. I always will.

You'll only attract sankes if you shut off your ability to identify sankes. You only make yourself vulnerable to sankes by not listening to your own good sense and inspiration.

What if I told you that the only thing that makes you vulnerable is believing you have no power? That you are powerful?

But my life proves otherwise.

Your life proves you can be knocked around and survive, which is one way you're powerful. Every upsetting event in your life was preceded by a gut feeling. Yes?

I suppose. Okay; yes. But I didn't act on it.

What if, from now on, you did listen to your gut sense? What if you did speak up?

I would be very powerful. I'd be like the Hoover Dam.

Do you know what the Hoover Dam does?

It converts the force of the water into electricity when water is released?

Exactly, and you can too. You can convert anything you perceive as negative energy into electricity to generate your own power.

I've gotten into a lot of trouble for knowing things I intuited.

But you've gotten into even more trouble ignoring your intuition, overruling what you knew, and dismissing your gut sense.

I didn't know how to handle the blowback of speaking up. I *was* powerless.

You're not powerless, you're not a victim, you're the Hoover Dam. You're a powerful energy detective. You decide who and what comes into your field of energy. When someone oversteps your boundaries, you can shake it off. Literally. You can move energy in, and you can move energy out.

Do you mean I can go out more and talk to people? I'm not defenseless?

No, you're not defenseless.

I can be myself? I don't need to hide?

You don't need to hide.

I like this. I can be upfront. I can offer my opinion whether anyone believes me or not.

Open the floodgates a bit at a time and celebrate. You're an energy detective, receptive and sheltered forever in my cave.

—⚊—

I start packing and neatly set my gifts on top so they don't get smushed.

Bedrock

I'm packed and ready to leave. I've been in a whirlwind since I woke up. I'm sleeping about five hours a night, which feels like a miracle. It also feels like cheating. I'm taking the medications the ER doc prescribed, as prescribed, but I worry I'll get addicted. My sponsor says otherwise, and I'm doing my best to believe her. She says healing is possible, but only if I get some sleep, eat well, and do what the doctor recommends.

I've staked out hotels in nearly every town between Phoenix and the north just in case I get an ocular migraine. I only plan to drive three hours a day, so I'm not a hazard to other drivers.

I look under the couch, in the closet, open and close each drawer, and check to make sure I packed my ratty but beloved robe, which usually hung on the back of the bathroom door. It's not there, and it wasn't there the latest two times I checked. I'm stalling, and there's nothing of mine left. I can't put off leaving any longer. Expect maybe a quick check-in with Cave Woman.

—⚊—

Dear Cave Woman,

I can't wait to see Cole, but I also don't want to leave my friends. Deciding to leave has been agonizing. I have friends here. I have a community. I'm not sure I have the tenacity to find another community. I still feel like I have a big target on my back that says: Victim Available.

You may not find another community right away. If not, keep looking. Get creative. You need to heal, and Cole needs healing, too. You will face challenges. What you need right now is a big dose of self-regard.

What size bottles does self-regard come in?

Every human is born with self-love. It never goes away. The Unreliable Narrator gets programmed by family, by the media, and by a misguided society that leaves people seeing themselves as helpless against perpetrators, which is just fine with all the thugs, bullies, and sankes of the world. It's time to let Sylvia be Sylvia.

I just don't want to run into any more sankes.

You will.

Then I'm staying here.

That won't help. Sankes are everywhere. You need to build your strength and gain self-regard for the challenges ahead no matter where you live.

I can't stop wondering if I'll get stuck in victim mode.

Your Survival Brain constantly scans for where you're being victimized. That's what it does. Going forward, don't mistake being a victim for the mere awareness of danger.

Okay, I hear you. I just don't want to act like a victim at all. That would be embarrassing. If anyone asked, I'd never admit I see myself as a victim. It's awfully dramatic.

When you were little, you needed to play the defeated victim to stay safe. Now, you're worried about appearing helpless and being vulnerable to sankes. This is progress.

Ensuring people think they're helpless makes them dependent and controllable. That's how patriarchy operates. See victimhood for what it is; an old protective pattern you no longer need.

How horrific. I've judged other people who seem to play the victim. I've judged them harshly. I hate myself. I feel disgusting. I'm a victim for seeing myself as a victim.

Hating yourself is one way to keep the pattern of victimization running. It's time to stop hating yourself. You're about to drive a car for several days, not long after a trip to the emergency room with impaired vision and difficulty speaking. We need to step up your lessons and do it quickly. I hate to tell you this, but we have no time to waste. You need to love yourself.

Then I'm doomed to be a victim because loving myself is impossible. I'll have to leave my car here and grab a bus or a plane.

You can do this. You were programmed to turn on yourself through repetition. One way you can cut away all those thick vines is by constantly repeating that you love yourself.

Hey, wait. I just need to repeat it, not necessarily believe it?

You know, you're right. Good thought. You don't need to believe it. You just need to repeat the phrase. You can love the organs of your body, the tissues and veins, each emotion, and each hive member. Your Survival Brain and Creative Genius will do the rest. Your mother's love continues to buoy you up. I'm with you, loving you, and supporting you always. You have a wealth of love vibrating from the core of your Creative Genius, from the soul of every animal who ever lived. By repeating "I love me" as a constant mantra, the old Survival Brain roots and vines will shrivel up and make room for more love to bloom.

Love is where you stand in order to pull others up. You can't preach love while standing in self-hatred.

I don't know. I'll need to give this some thought. Hey, wait. Weren't you're going to teach me a way to counterbalance my emotions?

Let's try counterbalancing. That would be a good one for your drive.

As you feel emotions about the past or worry about the future, identify the emotion—

And feel it?

Naturally.

And then?

Find some antonyms and feel those counterbalancing emotions, too.

For example?

When you think about whether Cole really wants you back, what emotion do you feel?

I feel unsure. I feel it in my forehead, heavy and furled.

Now find and feel the counterbalance. Can you feel confident?

Nah.

How about reliable?

I'm definitely more reliable than before recovery. Yes, I can feel reliable. I feel slightly taller and surer. I like this antonym game. What other words are a counterbalance for unsure?

Let's see. How about persistent?

Persistence is my favorite. I like how I can feel persistent without the pressure of having to be brave. Brave seems hard. Persistence feels light yet still has some forward motion.

What else?

When you find yourself ruminating about the awful job, what emotion do you feel?

Dread. I dread remembering. I dread running into more sankes. I dread facing Cole after being such a fool.

What's the opposite of dread?

Comfort?

Can you feel comfort? Can you remember a time you felt comforted?

I'm sure there are many times I felt comforted. I just can't feel comforted right now.

That's fine. Let's keep playing. How about lucky?

I am lucky. I'm lucky I get to make amends for leaving Maddy. I think I'll volunteer at the animal shelter and pet the kitties. I'm lucky to be in recovery. Lucky feels buoyant and a little sad.

And how does sad feel?

Like an old friend who's fine just hanging out with no need to explain anything.

Well said. Now get going.

I zip up my backpack with the notebook inside. I leave the key on the coffee table and shut the door behind me.

I walk tall and savor my transient home in the desert for the last time. Gloomy thoughts—to put it charitably—descend through me like a penny thrown in a deep ocean. Fears hits my stomach so hard, I cough. I break out in a sweat and test my vision. Is it usually this bright, or am I in trouble again? My head performs a little pirouette, and my heart reels. Out of desperation, I say to myself, "I love me," and the dizziness stops. I continue to repeat, "I love me," as I get in my car, drive through light traffic, and out of Phoenix for the last time.

Twenty minutes later, the early morning sweet-orange sunrise brightens the happy saluting cacti. I'm not feeling bright or sunny.

With each repetition of "I love me," my heartache grows about leaving the city I love. I cry big, gulping, snotty tears. It's not a picturesque goodbye. The large pile of wadded-up tissues expands next to the small cooler on the passenger-side floor. About an hour into the drive, I stop to use the bathroom and buy another box of tissues. I open the hatchback and dig around for a trash bag and fill it with my slimy wet tissues.

I refill my metal water bottle and open one of the green juices my friend supplied me with at my going away party. For my health and continued healing, they'd said. I'm worried I'll drink again without my support team, and my stomach spirals, and I start again: I love me, I love me, I love me.

As I repeat the mantra, I don't think about much, which is unusual for me. I'm surprised when I pull into the first scheduled hotel for this trip. The hotel is on an Indian reservation, and I'm embarrassed to remember sneaking in wine the last time I was here.

As I'm checking in, the hotel clerk says, "There's a pool if you'd like to swim."

I turn my head toward the courtyard and a large inviting pool. "I would, actually.

Thank you."

"You look surprised. Do you like to swim?"

"I do, and I'd love to go for a swim. I'm surprised because I thought I'd be more tired than I am," I say, not bothering to explain further, and we smile at each other anyway.

"Some local kids are dancing tonight here in the lobby. Maybe you'd be up for that too?" he politely asks. "It should be fun for everyone."

"I love things that are fun for everyone." We smile at each other again as I hand over my credit card and get my room key.

Souvenir

The pool has a turtle mosaic that undulates as I push off and glide under the water. I watch as the turtle and I gently undulate in tandem. For the second time today, and the second time in my adult life, I lose track of time. The water and the turtle and I roll along like the best of friends, reunited after a long absence.

I see a galaxy of purple and dark blue stars trailing across my body when I close my eyes.

A thought pops to mind. I know what this is. I've drowned, and I'm having a near-death experience. I startle and feel a wave of panic. I pull my head above the water and gasp for breath. I move toward the side and pull myself clumsily out of the water and onto the cement. I hit with a thud and know I've bruised a few ribs.

I sit by the pool wrapped in a large towel and breathe into the panic. The panic dissipates so quickly, I laugh at myself and realize I'm leaving a place but not running away. I tip my water bottle toward the turtle. I feel a sense of wellbeing, which wasn't at all how I expected this day to turn out. I left my notebook in my room and leave the pool to write Cave Woman.

Dear Cave Woman,

Saying "I love me" lost its impact fairly quickly today. But the antonym game was a blast. I'd have a memory or resentment come up, feel the emotion, but then I'd explore antonyms. My whole being felt a little different each time I evoked contrary emotions. Counterbalancing didn't make the original emotion disappear completely, but I felt more emotionally balanced.

You get to choose what works best. Well done. Rest your eyes for a bit, okay?

I will.

—⁓—

Equus Coaching

Odell grew up with horses. She told me the horses saved her from the abuse she suffered from humans. During my final weeks in Phoenix, we'd talked about post-traumatic stress. Odell thinks everyone with an addiction also has PTS.

She'd recommended I work with an Equus coach. Odell said the horses taught her how to rely on her instincts and clear the residue from past trauma.

The Equus coach Odell recommended in Arizona was booked, but there's one in the north, about four hours from my final destination. I scheduled a session for the third day of my trip and reserved the guest cottage for the night.

I'm taking a different route back to Cole than the one we traveled before. The alpine scenery is gorgeous if you like that type of thing. On the second night, I stay in a boxy hotel with small rooms, and I realize I only have about a two-hour drive to get to the ranch where I'll meet my Equus coach and, I imagine, a horse or two.

Before I leave the hotel, I bookmark a website of recovery meetings I'll be attending in the town I thought I'd left forever. The butterflies in my stomach are acting like I'm seeing Cole today. I remind them we'll see him tomorrow.

My car hugs curves as I approach the mountain town that will be my home for the night. I reach the top of each rise and briefly become a pilot, sailing the magnified sky. I touch down and find the ranch next to a low, wide creek. Dozens of cottonwood trees protect the house, barn, and guesthouse. My heart kicks when I remember how much my mom loved cottonwoods. I park near the guesthouse, a restored brick building. I can tell by the sandblasted brick it was recently refurbished. Ranches, barns, and farm animals are about as foreign to me as Jupiter. But with Odell's encouragement, I'm open to working with the horses. I'm glad I didn't have time to think this through. Horses are big.

Jeslyn, the ranch owner and my Equus coach for the day, stands in the doorway and greets me with a hopeful smile. She gives me a tour of the original barn, now a newly renovated guesthouse. In contrast to the old west exterior, the exposed brick and cast-iron railings made me think of a New York City loft. Maybe someday Cole and I could return and stay for a few days.

I bring in my overnight bag and use the bathroom, then Jeslyn asks if I'm ready. I tell her I'm excited.

We talk about my goals for the day and what to expect.

"I'm new to recovery," I say, figuring if I want help, I might as well be honest. "I understand working with the horses can help heal some of the reasons I may have started drinking in the first place."

"Well, first I want to say congratulations. I have family members in recovery. I know how hard that can be." I appreciate her honesty and start to tear up. I appreciate how difficult it must be to care about someone with an addiction. "I hope they didn't give you too much trouble on their way to recovery?" I offer.

"Fair to middling," she quips.

I want to say I didn't make trouble, but that's not true since we're being honest. I may not have encountered cops or judges, but I managed to cause trouble in my own way. I think about Maddy and Cole and our phantom trip to save the world. My focus dims.

Jeslyn watches me start to fade away and brings me back with a question. "Do you communicate with animals?" she asks.

I'm too surprised to lie and say, "Sometimes I think they talk to me, and I see animals when I close my eyes." I feel my face turn red.

"That's a good thing. No need to be embarrassed," Jeslyn reassures me.

"Oh, good. I thought maybe I was nuts," I say and look away.

Jeslyn kindly changes the subject. "Are you afraid of horses?" she asks.

"No. I did some trail rides as a kid, nothing fancy. The horses seemed pretty disinterested in humans."

"Well, we'll see," she says and leads me through a field of tall grass, rich with the smell of aged manure and warm hay, toward the round pen.

As we walk, she explains that the horses are keenly attuned to our state of being and our intentions. "We are predators, and as prey animals, horses have to be acutely alert to any danger we might pose."

We sit on a rough-sawn wooden bench by the round pen, and she introduces me to Glory, a chestnut stunner with eyes and ears pointed toward me like searchlights.

Jeslyn gives me a stiff coiled rope and instructions on how to command the horse to follow my lead. I tell her I'm ready. Jeslyn opens the gate, and I step in. I shyly bow my head to not spook Glory and walk forward.

Standing in the center of the round pen, I lift the rope to shoulder height and silently beg the ample copper horse to please walk, run, or trot. Anything, please. He stands stock-still. I lower my head in defeat, and my shoulders slump forward.

Jeslyn, standing just outside the gate, urges me to try again.

I attempt to become as serene as Snow White, picturing birds landing on my arms and gracing me with a crown of wildflowers. Glory blinks his eyes and swats flies away with his tail. I lower my head again and let the rope fall against my legs.

"Okay, come on out," suggests Jeslyn.

She offers me water from a cooler, and we sit in the shade on the bench. I've never spent much time around horses, but I like everything about this place.

"I notice you're timid."

"That obvious, huh?" I ask.

We both laugh.

"I was outgoing when I was very young. I'd talk with people wherever we went. It horrified my older sister. But then I became terribly shy at around age seven. Ever since, I've felt almost embarrassed to be alive."

"There were several traumas in your life. Tell me where I'm wrong?"

"You're not wrong."

"Did you feel timid in the round pen?"

"Very. But I tried to feel peaceful."

"Do you feel peaceful?"

"Not in the least little bit. I'm mad. Really mad."

"Good. That gives us something to work with. Horses are prey animals. They know if you're not honest about your feelings. Horses assume you're up to no good If you're hiding your feelings. For their own safety."

Standing once again in the center of the round pen, I wonder if my sharp anger could hurt this enormous and proud horse. I wave the rope a few more times, but he doesn't budge. He snorts and shakes his head. I return to the wooden bench and talk with Jeslyn.

She says, "For a horse to want to be a part of your herd, and essentially that's what you're asking, the horse has to know that you trust yourself, that you're honest about your feelings. If you don't have your best interest at heart, how can the horse trust you to look after his?"

"You mean I should be selfish?" I ask.

"Yes, in a sense. If you're busy worrying about what others think or what they did or didn't do, you're not paying attention to any possible threat from predators. That could be deadly."

I embarrassingly admit my true concern. "And I won't hurt him with all this anger I have inside?"

"Not at all. Glory knows what you're feeling already, but he'll only trust you if you're transparent about how you feel. Clarity is calming. Clarity is good for the herd. Transparency makes you trustworthy."

I reenter the center of the round pen.

I tune into my body. The anger feels like a lead ball with dull spikes inside my throat. I let the anger spread, and it drops to my chest with a heavy thud. The rage is ignited, and like lasers, the anger shoots out of my toes and fingertips. I look at a boulder by the creek and wonder if I could cut it in half by just pointing a finger.

I walk in a small circle in the center of the round pen. I hear another horse in the barn hit its hoof against a stall. Butterflies spin and dip toward the creek. The rush of the water becomes raucous. The birds take turns singing, politely speaking one at a time. A dog rolls around the dirt under a dried-up grey wagon entangled in weeds. I smell leather and hay and fresh-cut grass.

I even my eyes with Glory's. My back straightens, and the tension along my spine eases. My hand loosely grips the stiff roll of rope. I lift it about a foot from my body. Glory walks. I pick up my pace, feel the anger, and lift the rope height. Glory begins to trot. I pick up my pace and direct a surge of anger from my shoulders toward the Earth. Glory runs.

On a whim, I turn in the other direction. Glory turns and follows my lead. I stand in the center and point with the rope, directing him when to run, walk, and turn around. The anger moves in rhythm with my pulse. My rage feels powerful. I'm elated.

I merely think the word "stop" and Glory stops on a dime. I stand straight. I don't look at Jeslyn. I don't need to. We're all tuned to the same channel.

This is power. This is connection. This is love.

I look back at Glory and think "run" and to my everlasting amazement, he halls off and runs once more.

A wave of contentment pours through me. With the rope still at my side, I think the word "walk" and Glory walks. I think "Jeslyn" and we walk side by side to the gate. We contentedly stand in a circle. I think about the weeks and months ahead. I think briefly about how I'll be able to handle emotions without a horse and Jeslyn to guide me, and the worry sinks to my stomach. Then, quicker than I can lift my arms to protect myself, Glory takes his enormous head and wallops me in the gut.

I stumble back and laugh, surprised but impressed.

"Are you okay?"

"Yes, I'm fine. I started to feel anxious. I think he was telling me to trust my gut and not worry so much?"

"I think you're correct. All worry does is keep you from noticing whatever is happening right now. Whether it's a threat or a deep joy."

"Good point. Smart horse. Can I take him home with me?"

We laugh again, and a few tears roll down my cheeks. We're quiet as Glory gently nuzzles the crook of my neck, and I'm flooded with goosebumps.

As we walk back toward the guesthouse, a car pulls up next to mine. I'm surprised but oddly not shocked to see Cole get out of the passenger side. Cole's brother-in-law waves from the driver's side. I had a feeling I might see Cole today. The landscape came alive earlier, and now I feel a solid part of it, too. Whole and buzzy. I'm looking forward to getting this man I love alone.

Cole's brother-in-law revs his car as he backs out and shouts out the window, "Got to get to a meeting here in town. Good to see you. We're glad you're back."

He winds down the driveway as I shout, "Thanks for the delivery."

Cole smiles. I smile, too.

Jeslyn and I keep walking toward Cole, and I say, "After today, after working with you and Glory, I'm ready to be a partner again. I don't feel like I'll explode on him at any minute."

"You might want to tell Cole what you just told me," Jeslyn suggested.

"What a great idea. Thank you. Funny how working with an animal made me fit to be around humans again."

"I do believe animals give us back our humanity. I hope you come back again."

"I'm already counting the days," I say as I reach Cole and wrap my arms around him.

I let go even as he extends his hand to Jeslyn and introduces himself.

Jeslyn says, "Come by the barn in the morning. I'll be there bright and early. Sil has a new friend I think you'd like to meet."

"I appreciate that. Sil looks happy."

I smile and shake my head yes and say, "I'll tell you all about my new friends."

I open my arms and give Jeslyn a hug and thank her again for an amazing day.

Cole and I walk inside, and we sit on the couch. "I'm kind of sweaty, and I smell like horses. I'm going to take a shower, but first…" tears fill my throat, "I want to thank you for a thousand second chances. It couldn't have been easy."

"You did the hard work. All I did was dream this day real."

Acknowledgments

Thank you to my book coach, Nicole Criona, for helping me find the power of writing as medicine.

Thank you to every emotion, from apathy to euphoria, for their tenacious guidance.

Thank you to all the authors who have changed my life. Starting with Dr. Howard Schubiner, Karla McLaren, and Peter A. Levine. The list is long and ever-growing, which I continue on my website: dearcavewoman.com

What's Next

Dear Cave Woman,

Now what?

The healing continues.

Forever? You mean I'm not done?

Healing is a lifelong adventure It'll be worth it, I promise.

What'll we talk about?

Resolving pain and navigating life as a high perceiver.

Okay, okay, now I'm interested.

For updates on offerings, new releases,
and more acknowledgments, please visit:
dearcavewoman.com